Practise Happiness

The Energy of Life

Justine Lamboley

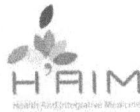

H'AIM
Health And Integrative Medicine

Practise Happiness

The Energy of Life

Justine Lamboley

First Printing, 2015

ISBN 978-0-9934240-2-1

H'AIM
Health And Integrative Medicine
152-160 City Road
EC1V 2 NX LONDON (UK)

For general information on our other products and services, you can contact us as contact.haim@haim.academy. For more information visit our website www.haim.academy

Contents

Foreword

Justine Lamboley presents in this book a panoramic vision, a synthesis and accurate information that invite the reader to choose and even to commit to fully experience a true yet accessible health.

The question which arises is: "Have we decided to do something for ourselves?" I like this distance that the author leaves us. This space allows us to appreciate that we are still the masters of our choices.

She gives us concrete possibilities to restore and maintain our potential of qualitative energy. This energy enables our body to regulate itself and therefore to prevent dysregulations and the development of diseases.

Of course, she goes back to the fundamentals: food, oxygenation, hydration, and elimination. But if they are unavoidable, they are nevertheless not sufficient. Because health is the expression of a unity Body and Spirit, the manifestation of two complementary energies which are in constant interaction.

We understand that health is built on a state of inner peace, of serenity, that is to say the emotional harmony and the quality of thought.

This verticality emphasised here by the author is mandatory. She has the boldness to invite anyone seeking health to open a space for prayer. Does this mean that we must open ourselves up to a simple spirituality where happiness can be the cure of all suffering?

We find here the tradition of Man between heaven and earth, the Body-Spirit unity of a man in his verticality, connected to himself and connected to the universe . . . Justine dares to share this experience. The author provides it to us with clarity and simplicity.

It fulfills here the dream of every human being: HEALTH—LONGEVITY—HAPPINESS AND SHARING.

Dr Somchay INTHAVONG
MD, Psychoanalyst, Homeopath
International guest speaker
Based in Aix en Provence (France)
Geneva (Switzerland), Vientiane (Laos)

Introduction

Why Is the Way We Live So Important?

Life is the most amazing present of nature, but all too often, we miss the privilege of enjoying it, preoccupied as we so easily are by all kinds of activities in our daily life. It has been the force of life that has been the engine that brought bacteria, vegetal elements, animals, and human beings to the earth. The vital force of life also allows children to grow, our bodies to heal, plants or trees that have been cut off to grow again through the emergence of small buds . . . Nature brings back to life what appears dead with a fabulous energy.

Our body is a fantastic machine that has all kinds of sophisticated processes to repair itself. The latest scientific discoveries even show us that cells that are cancerous can revert and repair themselves.[1] However, when too many destructive factors are around us, the capacity of our body to maintain perfect health and repair itself when needed is hindered.

We are overwhelmed by the appearance of new illnesses. Every day, we see a drastic increase of what is now called "civilisation diseases". We hear that we should not eat this food as it causes cancer, or another food causes degenerative

---

[1] Bodin L. *Cancer, the paths towards healing (Revertant cells)* (Paris: Tredaniel, 2014), 20.

diseases. We hear that this fantastic regime will help us lose weight and enjoy vibrant health, before being debunked a few months later by competitors who offer a better regime.

We hear that our air is polluted, our water is polluted, that electromagnetic fields are disturbing our health, and that we have heavy metals in our teeth . . . All this makes it quite difficult in the end to know what we should eat and how we should live. Many companies and purveyors of "happiness" take advantage of this confusion to cash in on millions by selling miraculous products that don't work.

I do not intend to give miraculous recipes for happiness and vibrant health, but I know that by using a few practical keys to provide good food for your body, mind, and spirit, you will quickly see the positive effects of your practise to improve your life. Life is simple, but we often miss the simplest things because they are not complicated, and we think that it should be complicated to work out. We think that happiness cannot be accessed easily or otherwise everyone would practise it . . . The truth is, life is easy, but few people around the globe can access a prosperous life based on and attuned to nature's laws.

Degenerative diseases, where good cells die one after another; cancer, where healthy cells get damaged and start proliferating in an uncontrollable way; immune diseases, where the cells of the body turn themselves against the body, might only be a mirror of the society in which we live . . . Everything goes faster and faster; development and growth have developed activities that are destroying the earth; many technical innovations have developed so much that they are unmanageable, a bit like these diseases affecting a body that is confused about how to find the way to heal itself.

And in a world where there is seemingly more than enough abundance, there is more and more structural poverty, which is a parallel to the food that we eat, which is more and more abundant but is poor in terms of the essential minerals and vitamins it brings to the body. We fail to have the necessary nutrients, and we eat too much fat and sugar, which destroy our body . . . We also have instant access to information, we study, travel, do multiple activities more than ever before, but we often lose the connection to ourselves and the inner peace we are looking for.

But life gets simple once we become connected to ourselves, to nature, and to the vibrations of the earth. The more we become aligned with this vibration, the better we feel.

Stress and chronic acidosis

Most people in Western societies suffer from acidosis,[2] which means that we have too much acidity in our tissues and body. Stress and processed food are the main reasons for this acidosis. It affects all our eliminating organs, liver, intestine, and kidneys, but also sometimes our skin or breathing abilities.

Stress and negative emotions produce an acidic pH in our tissues, which will try to find alkaline minerals stored in our body to reduce this acidity . . . using vital resources. The body as a result absorbs fewer and fewer nutrients, the

---

[2] We are talking here of acidosis in its naturopathic acceptance, which relates to an acidosis of tissues. This is not a blood acidosis, which often requires an emergency medical intervention.

energy produced by cells decreases, and the body struggles to repair damaged cells. If we feed our body with more sweeteners, coffee, beer, cigarettes, cow milk, cheese, ice creams, etc., we increase this acidity. Stress causes acidity and acidity causes stress. It is a vicious circle that maintains itself in a loop.

Acidosis brings different disorders—the person might feel tired, irritated, have difficulties to control emotions, feel cold, have brittle hair, often dandruff, allergies are developing, eczema or skin disorders can appear, intestines are not working properly with either constipation or diarrhoea, immunity is affected, menstrual periods are painful for women, and fertility is affected. People who are stressed and do a lot of intellectual work are particularly affected by acidosis.

By adapting the diet, first by reducing this chronic stress, the quality of life can be improved. We have to understand that our body is not a machine that has to work the way our modern society wants it to work.

We have to be aware that when our body does not function as it should, it gives us alarms (such as pain) to signal that something is wrong. Most of the time, we take medicine to stop the pain. We are like a driver who sees a red button flashing on the dashboard of the car but hits the command board until the red signal switches off. What will certainly happen is that the car will break down and the driver will have to change the engine or big pieces, which are now broken.

If he/she had first taken into considerations these lights and taken the car to a mechanic, it is likely that the mechanic would have stopped the problem and repaired the car much quicker and for a lower price. Maybe it was just about adding a bit of oil or water. By looking much closer at our body and trying to find the real cause of a disorder, we might fix the problem in a natural way, which will enable us to lessen or forgo an allopathic treatment.

But also we have to understand that our body is connected to a mind and a spirit. If we receive an emotional shock, or if we entertain ourselves with extremely negative thoughts, these thoughts will decrease our vital energy and they might cause an illness. Many researchers have shown that cancer, for instance, is triggered by an emotional shock. It is not the cause, but it triggers the illness to wake up and develop.

According to the part of the body, we will know what kind of conflict has caused the cancer to develop. In the case of breast cancer, whether it is left or right, it is a conflict with (or for) the partner or with the children. You might have heard, for instance, that a friend who is divorcing developed breast cancer at the same time . . . the shock of divorce is sometimes so strong for a woman that it might trigger the cancer to develop. Colon cancer relates to something the person did not forgive, did not digest or let go. Lung cancer is linked to the fear of dying.

Why is this so important?

Our emotions and thoughts are important and the more positive thoughts we have, the higher our energetic vibrations are. With the constant increase of the earth vibrations, we notice easily that people who eat industrial food, feed their mind with negativity (TV is an example), have their vibration decreasing. It might well mean a decrease in immunity but also a state of unwellness or mild depression.

We know also that refined and processed food causes an excess of sugar and oils in the body, causing all kinds of intestinal problems, such as the Candida albicans, pinworms, and intestinal dysbiosis. Our belly is our second brain, where all information is stored in addition to emotions. This imbalance in the intestine has a strong impact on our psychological and emotional health. By exchanging the bacteria of the microbiota of two mice, one became aggressive, the other one peaceful, when it was the other way around before the switch of the bacteria present in the intestinal flora.[3]

Meat and animal proteins were given in ancient times to fabricate warriors. It fosters aggressivity. Cereals, on the contrary, were mainly eaten in Europe by poor people who had to be submissive to their sovereign. We now know that yogurt contains bacteria that help people to relax and be more peaceful. If we look at the way of eating in different cultures, we often notice that the higher caste, or spiritual caste, does not eat meat and animal products. The Egyptian priests, the Brahmans, and the Buddhists in general are vegetarians. It is thought that avoiding meat raises spiritual energies.

So the way we eat, the way we think, we talk, we live, the place we live in, especially with the increasing disturbance of electromagnetic fields (Wi-Fi, antennas, electric high-voltage

---

[3] Collins S et al. The adoptive transfer of behavioural phenotype via the intestinal microbiota: Experimental evidence and clinical implications. *Current opinion in microbiology* 16, 3 (June 2013): 240–245.

lines) added to geobiological disorders (if your house is over a telluric chimney, vortex, or a river) completely changes your life.

We can be miserable or prosperous in all its terms. These three parameters: (1) diet (ahara), (2) lifestyle (vihara), and (3) having a peaceful mind (manovya para) are the basis of Indian medicine (Ayurveda). Once our vital energy flows freely, our mind is calm and peaceful, our soul goes on its path of life . . . and we can live without illness or suffering, going towards an unlimited joy and infinite happiness.

What I want for you now is to understand that whatever we have been taught, we are the actors of our life. We might not have all the same resources, but we can make the most with what we have to enjoy our life in the best way possible.

Chapter 1

Food for My Body

Diet is the number one risk factor for death in most regions of the world, except for some parts of Oceania and Sub-Saharan Africa.[4] First causes of death in the United States are heart disease, cancer, chronic respiratory diseases, and stroke. Three of them are greatly linked to an unhealthy diet and lifestyle. Two-thirds of Americans are obese (61 percent); 66 percent of Emirati men and even 80 percent of Egyptian women are suffering from obesity.[5] Among the Saudi population, the prevalence of diabetes increased from 10.6 percent in 1989 to 32.1 percent in 2009.[6] One out of three American children born in 2000 will develop diabetes

---

4 Institute for Health Metrics and Evaluation' (IHME). Global Burden Disease (GBD) 2010 study.

5 Caroll L. Obesity in the Gulf: Disturbing new survey. *The National, UAE* (29 May 2014).

6 Alharbi NS, Almutari R, Jones S, Al-Daghri N, Khunti K, and De Lusignan S. Trends in the prevalence of type 2 diabetes mellitus and obesity in the Arabian Gulf States: Systematic review and meta-analysis. *Diabetes research and clinical practice* 106, 2 (November 2014): e30–e33.

during his or her lifetime.[7] All these worrying figures show that eating can kill us and make us extremely sick. However, it does not have to be that way as physical food is the most important element of good health and well-being.

In antique times, food was considered the main medicine: "Let food be thy medicine and medicine be thy food", states the famous saying of Hippocrates. We now hear everywhere "you are what you eat" and we only grasp the meaning of the sentence once we start shifting towards a healthier diet as a lighter, greener, and healthier diet leads to physical and psychological drastic changes in our life.

Culinary habits are one of the most significant parts of our social identity and sense of belonging to a community. Eating brings essential energy to our body, it helps our body and organs to function, and it supports the healing process of our body when it gets sick. It also brings pleasure and satisfaction that is best shared around the family or community table. Food habits are the last identifying marker that immigrants retain, whereas language, clothes, and religion are often adapted to the environment they are living in from the first generation.

For instance, it is not rare to see descendants of 1920s Italian immigrants to New York City still eating only Neapolitan and Mediterranean cuisine even one century after their ancestors moved from the old continent. The same often applies for

---

[7] Venkat Narayan KM, Boyle JP, Thompson TJ, Sorensen SW, and Williamson DF. Lifetime risk for developing diabetes mellitus. *JAMA* 290 (2003): 1884–1890.

Chinese, Lebanese, Middle Eastern Jewish immigrants who have passed on their cuisine from one generation to the next, even in the most remote places of the world. Therefore our eating habits are deeply rooted in ourselves and it is hard for us to change the unhealthy parts.

In addition, the development of fast foods, readymade meals, industrial and refined foods have deeply changed our diets. For many teenagers living in developed countries, lettuce and French fries are their main source of vegetables, leaving out essential nutriments from their diets. In general, we eat too many saturated fats and processed carbohydrates, too much salt, sugar, and animal protein, which leads to deadly diseases mentioned above but also to smaller annoying disorders, such as digestion and intestinal disorders, chronic fatigue, and joint pain to mention a few.

From hunting and picking fruits from trees, human beings are now mostly seating in front of a screen for long hours . . . therefore the amount of food and type of food should be adapted to their daily activities: seating at a desk with the air conditioner set up at 20 degrees Celsius might require less food intake than working in the construction sector in Alaska, for instance.

Various studies since the 1950s seem to indicate that the Mediterranean diet or Cretan regime increases life expectancy and reduces the risk of cardiovascular incidents, diabetes Type 2, and Alzheimer's diseases.[8] In this type of diet, the main oil consumed is olive oil, along with fruits, vegetables, and foods with a high amount of fibre. These are fostered whereas the consumption of meat and dairy products is more limited.

However, there are so many contradicting studies and books about various regimes and miracle diets (which all promise you to be beautiful and slim in a few weeks or erase all your health problems) that it is hard to know which one to choose. You will find in this book practical advice on which foods should be avoided and which nutriments should be fostered. But I tend to think that in the end, you should make your own personal diet by taking into account your body constitution, your level of vital energy, the place you live, and combine various recommendations to establish a healthy diet for your body with a healthy food for your mind, which will be explained in the next chapter. Also, you should remember that following a strict diet should be limited to a few weeks or months; it is not intended, as the word suggests, to be a lifelong way of eating.

---

[8] Keys A. Seven countries study (1958). Sofi F, Cesari F, Abbate R, Gensini GF, and Casini A. Adherence to Mediterranean diet and health status: Meta-analysis. *BMJ* (Clinical research ed.) (2008): 337–344.

10 main commandments for healthy food

1/ Do not cook or heat your meal in a microwave or pressure cooker. Prefer steam cooking, slow cooking, and a temperature below 80 degrees Celsius.

2/ Limit the consumption of readymade, industrial, and processed food.

3/ Limit your consumption of sugar (especially refined white or brown sugar). Prefer natural sugar contained in fruits.

4/ Limit your consumption of salt (readymade meals contain a lot of salt, for instance).

5/ Use cold pressed oils (olive, nuts, colza, corn, linen, almond, sunflower, if used cold. For cooking, use only olive oil).

6/ Eat more vegetables and fruits—whenever possible organic.

7/ Add more fibres and complete cereals (basmati or Thai plain rice, corn, quinoa, buckwheat).

8/ Reduce your consumption of gluten (mainly contained in wheat flour, white bread, pizzas, pasta, cakes).

9/ Reduce your consumption of meat (ban, if possible, pork and red meat, eat poultry without the skin).

10/ Eat more fish rich in omega 3 (prefer small fish, such as sardines, anchovies).

To cook or not to cook?

Eat raw vegetables whenever it is possible or cook them "al dente" to preserve the nutritive elements. Nowadays steam cookers are popular and although their quality vary greatly depending on their price and brand, you can find reasonably priced steam cookers, which will preserve the nutriments and remove many toxins, which are thrown away with the water that has been used in the lower pot.

If you are using a traditional oven, avoid covering your dish or wrapping the food with aluminium foil, as it is toxic for your body. Also, eating grilled meat on the barbecue might be tasty, but should not be eaten frequently as it produces polycyclic aromatic hydrocarbons (PAHs) and aromatic heterocyclic amines (AAH), which are carcinogens. But most important, do not use a microwave! Do not give it away, as it is a poisoned gift, just throw it away!

The microwave oven has been distributed since the 1960s around the Western world and many studies have shown its disastrous impact on living organisms. In Russia, microwaves were banned from importation in 1976 because of their negative consequences on health. In a microwave, electromagnetic waves generated by a high frequency transmitter (magnetron) penetrate the food and excite the molecules resulting in hyper-rapid oscillations. To make it simple, heating your food in the microwave is equivalent to experimenting with a kind of crazy shaking and irradiation of your food.

You might have heard about the experiment to grow two plants, one watered with tap water and one watered with water that had been heated in the microwave and cooled before being poured on the plant. Usually the plant watered with microwaved water died within six to nine days. Scientists have shown that the microwaves break the molecules of the food, remove all the vitamins, and generate free radicals. Food heated in the microwave loses 60 to 90 percent of its vital energy and accelerates the disintegration of aliments. This means that what you eat has lost almost all its nutritive qualities, not to mention that your stomach and intestines have to make an extra effort to digest and process the food.

Make an effort, cook your own meal

As we saw in the Introduction, our modern lifestyle does not allow us to spend a lot of time cooking and eating. But industrial foods and readymade meals are deprived of most of the nutritive elements contained in food and many added components are harmful. Just try to read all the components written on a frozen meal that you bought at the local supermarket. You will easily notice that you do not have most of these components in your kitchen.

Most restaurants now serve industrial reheated food, and I was astonished to see all my favourite dishes in one of my friends' catalogue for professionals of the catering industry. Because of the sanitary regulations and policies of reduced costs, most of the food served in collectives and hospitals is deprived of any nutritive elements, so it should be avoided whenever possible. If one of your relatives is staying in a hospital, you can smuggle in natural, complementary food and vitamins pills with the advice of an experienced naturopath.

Sugar is stronger than cocaine!

Are we all drug addicts, really? A French researcher undertaking research about drug addiction discovered that rats preferred water sweetened with sugar more than cocaine when given the two options.[9] The more we eat sugar, the more we need it. Have you ever felt a bit down with a craving for a big chocolate cake or sweets? Sugar has become so usual in our diet that avoiding eating it is a real challenge as Eve Schaub,[10] an American mother of two children showed

---

[9] Lenoir M, Serre F, Cantin L, and Ahmed SH. Intense sweetness surpasses cocaine reward. *PLoS ONE* 2, 8 (2007): e698.

[10] Schaub E. *Year of no sugar: A memoir* (2014). Sourcebook.inc.

when she tried to wean her family from artificial sugar for one year.

Sugar consumption has sharply risen since the nineteenth century and our body does not adapt as fast as our diet changes. For instance, people in France consumed 5 kg of sugar per year per inhabitant in 1850, whereas it reached 45 kg in 1965. The amount decreased to 35 kg per year per inhabitant in the 1990s with the figure quite stable since then.

The world consumption is 20 kg per inhabitant, on average, but people of Singapore eat 84.7 kg per inhabitant per year! Costa Ricans eat 51 kg/year, New Zealanders 48 kg/year, and the British 45 kg/year, whereas Italians eat only 7 kg/year and Russians 6 kg/year, so consumption varies greatly from one country to the next. The main intake of sugar is due to prepared dishes. From the 35 kg consumed/year/inhabitant in France, 25 kg originates from saccharose (which makes 70g/day), a kind of sugar that is incorporated in sweet products.

Therefore, as much as possible we should avoid readymade products and foster natural sugar. A study published in the Journal of Biological Chemistry[11] in December 2007 shows that sugar fosters the development of Alzheimer's disease. Also, it decreases the cerebral functions, especially for

---

[11] Cao D et al. Intake of sucrose-sweetened water induces insulin resistance and exacerbates memory deficits and amyloidosis in a transgenic mouse model of Alzheimer's disease. *Journal of biological chemistry* (December 14, 2007).

children who consume sodas and sweet drinks. Dr Scott Kanoski [12] who released a study in 2014 states that "consuming sugar-sweetened drinks is interfering with our brain's ability to function normally and remember critical information about our environment, at least when consumed in excess before adulthood".

Sugar consumption should be limited to three teaspoons per day for children, but they usually consume ten times more (34 teaspoons/ day) in the United States. A single 33 cl soda contains 6 teaspoons of sugar! If you have an overactive child, try to cut all sugar intake and you should see amazing results within one to two months!

People who drink light or diet drinks, or who add artificial sweetener to their coffee or tea, should absolutely ban it. These drinks are usually worse for their health than the normal drink. Many studies show that it increases the diabetes risk, and some studies shows that it is responsible for many brain degenerative cases.

In conclusion, absolutely avoid white sugar, which is 100 percent refined and was popularised in the nineteenth century after the English, and then the French with Napoleon, imposed a block making the arrival of sugar in Europe impossible.

---

[12] Kanoski SE, Konanur VR, and Hsu TM. Adolescent consumption of sugar-sweetened beverages impairs hippocampal-dependent learning. Annual meeting of the Society for the Study of Ingestive Behavior. 2014.

An engineer soon found a chemical process to extract sugar from the beetroot juice. That is how white sugar was born, deprived of its mineral salts, cellulose, and vitamins. This sugar hinders digestion, slows the intestines' work, and can cause caries and bone decalcification.

Brown sugar is nothing more than white sugar that has been coloured with caramel and has lost all its nutritive elements. Therefore you should use unrefined full cane sugar or honey whenever possible or buy natural sugars, such as agave or stevia syrup, or rapadura. Also, 100 grams of unrefined cane sugar contains 250 calories, whereas white sugar contain 400 calories for the same 100 grams . . . so definitely ban white sugar from your home.

If you can, it's better to eat fruits that contain natural sugar. Until recent times that was the only sugar intake that our ancestors had. Fruits should be best consumed as snacks between meals, as they contain simple sugars that are quickly digested, either two hours before your lunch, or four hours after your lunch. If you had lunch quite late (that is after 13.00), it is best to eat fruits half an hour before dinner. For people wishing to lose weight, never eat fruit after your dinner, as your body will store the sugar for the night. It is best to stop all food intake, especially sugar, after 20.00, which is becoming harder and harder in our modern society, where dinner has become the main meal of the day.

Reduce salt intake

Prepared and readymade meals contain a lot of salt and people also add more salt to their meals, which causes artery hypertension, cardiovascular diseases, osteoporosis, and also increases the risk of stomach cancer, among other dysfunctions. Therefore, when you are cooking, use only gray, unrefined salt, as it contains all the minerals necessary for intestinal absorption.

Also, you can buy Himalayan pink salt, which is extracted 400–700 meters under sea level and has not been affected by pollution. It is very rich in nutrients, such as iron, calcium, magnesium, and potassium, and helps the regeneration of blood in the body. It is also known for decreasing blood pressure, reducing symptoms of arthritis, helping the intestinal transit, and reducing aging signs. Also its vibration level is much higher than other salts. As it is quite expensive, you might want to only use it for some preparations and otherwise use various herbs and spices to add flavour to your cooking.

About meat and milk

Nowadays, most of our protein intake in developed countries comes from meat and dairy products, but that has not always been the case. In agricultural societies, meat intake per person was rarely higher than 5–10 kilos per year. Germans and English, for instance, consumed only 20 kilos of meat per capita in 1800. It reached 60 kilos by the beginning of the twentieth century and is now about 80 kg/ year/ capita. In France, a sharp increase occurred only after 1950, when the consumption was less than 50 kilograms and reached more than 100 kilos in the 2000s.

In Asian countries, the changes in the traditional diet, which is mainly vegetarian with meat representing only 10 percent of the food intake, have been drastic in the past 40 years. The official Chinese figures report that meat production per capita was only 11.2 kg/capita in 1975, compared to 25 kg by 1990 and nearly 50 kg 10 years later. But many rural families still cannot afford meat. In many poor countries around the world, meat is reserved for feasts and special events, which is in fact much healthier, provided that there are enough vitamins and nutrients in other food sources.

Moreover, the globalisation tends to bring standardised Western food to many countries that cannot afford organic, premium, free-range chicken, creating an industry that harms nature but also humans, contributing to foul the body with hormones, dioxin, and residues of vaccines. There are videos showing containers of chicken carcasses and wings being taken to the African market, selling the cheapest parts of the chicken containing the highest concentration of hormones, after Europeans have bought at a much higher price the legs and breasts. As we know, toxins are stocked in higher quantities in the chicken wings and skin, therefore you should prefer chicken legs and breasts from organic or at least free-air farms.

Pork and all its derivatives (chorizo, bacon, salami sausages, and other delicatessens) should remain exceptional. Red meat should also be avoided as much as possible and reduced to one portion per week. White meat can be consumed once or twice a week, and should be organic or from a local farmer who raises chicken outdoors. Intestinal transit takes three, four, or even five days with refined and greasy foods from animal origin, whereas it takes 12 to 24 hours with vegetarian food.

By eating less meat, not only will you feel lighter, but your intestinal transit will be made easier, you will sleep better, and you will feel more energetic. One interesting thing is that the more we eat meat, the more we crave for meat, the more it makes us feel heavy and tired, and the more we think that we should eat meat to regain energy, which is totally contrary to what is happening in our body. When we feel tired we should eat less caloric food or even do a mono-meal day (as explained later) to allow our body to regenerate and find its vital energy.

Another argument might convince meat lovers to lower their meat intakes, as a wide study conducted among Seventh-day Adventists, [13] an American church where alimentary restrictions include not eating pork and avoiding all meats, have an increased life expectancy of seven years. Another study conducted among university medical students in a Seventh-day Adventist university in Loma Linda, California, and another university in southern California showed that breast cancer is three times lower in the Adventist university population.[14] Also, mortality rates caused by breast cancer were much lower for Adventist women who were vegetarian in comparison to other California women.

Another piece of news: milk is bad for our health. Remember the advertising of our childhood with cows walking freely in nice Swiss mountains with healthy, pink-cheeked kids drinking fresh milk? The dairy industry has convinced us for years now, thanks to heavy lobbying and advertising, that milk and its derivatives bring calcium to children, helping them to grow faster, and protect old people from osteoporosis. But, cow milk is not made to be drunk all

---

13 Fraser G and Shavlik DJ. Ten years of life: Is it a matter of choice? *Archive of internal medicine* 161, 13 (2003): 1645–1652.

14 Quoted by Schaller T. *Meat and milk: Dangerous nutrients which destroy or health and planet* (Lanor edition, 2007).

lifelong in such high quantities as it is the case in our societies.

Yoghurts did not exist 50 years ago. My neighbour, who is 103 years old and belongs to the funding family of Renault's cars in France, ate her first yogurt when she was 40 years old! And although she comes from a privileged background, cheese and milk were not as widely consumed as is the case now and did not have at all the same taste according to her. Moreover, cow milk is designed at the origin to feed small veal with the necessary nutrients corresponding to veal, not a human baby.

Human beings are the only animals on the whole earth to drink milk of another species. A baby fed with cow milk does not have the same faeces as a baby fed by breastfeeding; one has putrefying faeces while the other one has fermenting faeces. Also, when a baby starts his life, his intestinal system is not complete until he reaches the age of three years old and is totally complete at seven. So the food you get as a baby and a child is extremely important to build the right kind of bacteria in your intestinal flora.

Cow milk, for instance, contains 300 times more casein than the mothering milk. Casein is a kind of strong glue that fouls your intestinal system. Studies conducted by Dr Colin Campbell show that casein is one of the most powerful stimulating factor of cancer cells at any stage of a cancer.

Also, drinking cow milk increases various health disorders, such as increased cholesterol, acne, eczema, gas, intestinal disorders, allergies, and triggers the occurrence of diabetes 1.[15] In a study published in September 2014, which was done over a 20-year period among 61,433 Swedish women, and 45,339 men,[16] it was shown that high milk consumption is associated with higher mortality and higher fractures. For instance, women who drink three or more glasses of milk per day had a relative risk of death, "90 percent higher," and the risk of hip fracture was "60 percent higher" compared to those who drank less than one portion of milk per day.

The lowest rate of hip fractures is found among people who eat little or no dairy foods (these people are on lower calcium diets), such as people from rural Asia and rural Africa.[17]

The idea that milk helps you fight osteoporosis and is good for bones thanks to the calcium it contains might be misleading, as calcium is also contained in vegetables, is better absorbed by our system that way, and vegetarians do not lack calcium despite not drinking milk.

Our body needs a special enzyme to digest milk, which is the chymosin or labferment. This enzyme is present in our body

---

15 Dahl-Jorgensen K, Joner G, and Hanssen KF. Relationship between cows' milk consumption and incidence of IDDM in childhood. *Diabetes care* 14 (1991): 1081–1083.

16 Michaëlsson K et al. Milk intake and risk of mortality and fractures in women and men: Cohort studies. *BMJ* 349 (2014).

17 Abelow B. Cross-cultural association between dietary animal protein and hip fracture: A hypothesis. *Calcific tissue international* 50 (1992): 14–28.

until we are three years old, disappears and returns when we get old, that is after 70 years old. Americans, after centuries of drinking litres of milk every day now have the chymosin enzyme all life long, but the United States is one of the only nations to have it. It means that for all other people, milk cannot be digested easily during most of our life, not to mention that 50 percent of adults in Europe are intolerant to lactase, which is contained in milk, the rates being even higher in Asia or in Arab countries where people do not have the necessary enzymes to help their body with the digestion of cow milk.

In many countries farmers have been forced to use lactation-stimulating hormones, the recombinant bovine growth hormone (rbGH), which increases the cow's milk production but gives frequent infections, skin problems that are treated with antibiotics, which are to be found in the milk we drink. The European Union has so far not authorised the growth hormone under the precautionary principle, but most of the milk drunk around the world is far from the idyllic picture of happy cows eating grass in a pollution-free field.

Cheese and butter are subject to many contradicting studies, but as derivatives of milk they should be avoided as much as possible and be replaced by goat cheese, as proteins of goat milk contain proportionately less casein, and the amino acid profile of goat milk is close to that of human milk. Also, it's better to use vegetal butter, which is rich in omega 3 and lowers the cholesterol intake compared to the usual cow butter. For those who want to limit their fat intakes, remember that 74 percent of the calories contained in cheddar cheese are from fat and 100 percent of the calories in butter.

Soy milk has been subject to much criticism in the past years (and other non-fermented soy products, such as tofu) because it contains phytoestrogens, but many articles refer to a single study done by the Weston A. Price Foundation. Asian women have consumed soy products for centuries, which seems to be one of the factors of the limitation of breast cancer spread in these countries. Also, soy products, if consumed moderately, help to reduce the cholesterol rate. Therefore, unless you are facing thyroid issues, occasionally drinking soy milk might not be harmful, although you can definitely prefer rice milk, almond milk, oat milk (if you are not eating gluten-free) or coco milk.

In the end, proteins, whether vegetal or animal, must cover 12 to 15 percent of our food intake. They are important as they bring us essential amino acids. But you should choose carefully this protein intake. If you are vegetarian, you will need to mix and match cereals, legumins, and dry fruits to have a balanced input of those amino acids that are so useful to transport vitamins and nutrients.

Gluten free

Eating gluten free is spreading quickly around the world, especially since famous athletes have gone on gluten-free diets, such as the world's number one Serbian tennis player Novak Djokovic, 2013 Wimbledon winner Andy Murray, or French tennis player Jo-Wilfried Tsonga. According to the New Yorker magazine (2014), one third of Americans try to eliminate gluten from their diets.

Gluten comes from the Latin and means "glue". When glutenin and gliadin come into contact it forms a bond, an elastic membrane that is used by the food industry to link ingredients to one another. It is present in wheat, oat, rye, barley, bread, pizza, pasta, cakes, readymade meals, beer, soy sauce—30 percent of products found in the local supermarket contain gluten!

If eating gluten free requires a bit of organisation, especially in countries where it is quite uncommon to have gluten-free products, you quickly manage to eat outside without too much trouble. Usually Asian restaurants serve meals with a rice base, which makes things easier—provided that the chef doesn't add readymade sauces and gravies full of gluten. Potatoes and French fries are also an option, although fries are an unhealthy version of the latter.

Coeliacs, who are allergic to gluten, represent only 1 percent of the population, but one out of five persons is now intolerant to gluten, often without knowing it. The symptoms are usually eczema, gas, irritable bowel, strong pain in the stomach after eating, depression, and fatigue. Most of us have one of these symptoms, so would it mean that we are all allergic to gluten? In fact, the combination of a modern lifestyle with food different from what we ate 10,000 years ago, before the agricultural systems started to exist, seems to be responsible for this discomfort and these symptoms, but gluten is definitely making our digestion slower and more difficult, and its intake should therefore be reduced.

All the people around me who have taken off gluten out of their diets have seen spectacular results. My sister does not have animal hair and pollen allergies anymore, while her partner has seen a great improvement in his digestion and intestinal transit. Many premenopausal or menopausal women have seen hot flashes disappear totally once they stopped eating gluten.

I saw on multiple occasions eczemas vanishing and I found a great improvement of my energy level. I was always tired, always had a stone in my stomach after eating pizza or a big sandwich and all these symptoms disappeared within three weeks of a totally gluten-free diet. And usually after six months to one year of gluten abstinence, it is possible to introduce it again, from time to time a cake or piece of bread, without feeling any discomfort.

However, what makes things more complicated than it appears is the fact that gluten is not always responsible for these symptoms and discomfort. We have to know that the wheats that were used in the past have been modified over time and are not absorbed any more by our body. The wheat we had in 1850 has nothing to do with the wheat currently available in supermarkets, although it is now trendy to offer old wheat, such as the T65, until T145, which are unrefined wheats. Some people tolerate this wheat better and do not need to go on a gluten-free diet.

Also, organic wheat is not treated by pesticides for its conservation and is therefore better for health. Most small bakers do not use organic wheat as it perishes in less than three weeks and attracts all kind of rodents and insects. Also, most of the cereals we are eating are imported and transported by cargos directly in the hold of the ship.

To protect it from rodents and fungus, cargos are sprayed with pesticides, like bromomethyl, which is one of the main cause for professional illnesses among dockers who are unloading the ships. As a consumer of wheat, we are not as much exposed as dockers but we might still wonder about the effect these cereals have on our health. Therefore, I would advise that whether you decide to go gluten-free or eat wheat-based meals, it is essential to buy local organic wheats.

Is orange juice really good for our health?

The image of a perfect and healthy breakfast automatically goes together with a fresh glass of orange juice. A study conducted in France revealed that French people drink 27 litres of orange juice per year per inhabitant, and its consumption has been multiplied by seven times during the past 20 years. Drinking orange juice for breakfast is quite a new habit in Western societies and is far from being a good source of vitamins and nutrients.

First, concentrated juices and nectars are not real juice, in the sense that nectars often contain only 5 percent of fruit in the beverage. The rest is water, added sugar, and synthetic vitamin C. Nectars and concentrated juices actually contain more sugar than sodas and are deprived from natural vitamins, which have evaporated with the heat during the dehydrating process!

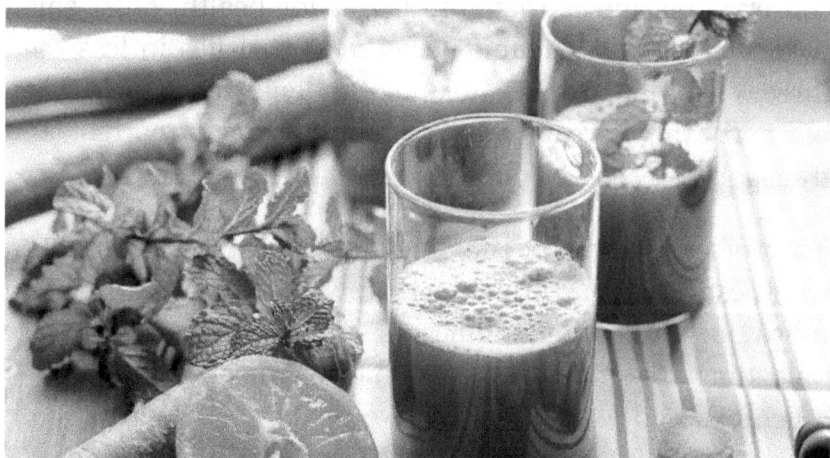

If you buy 100 percent fruit juice, you are drinking a healthier product, but vitamins are long gone by the time you drink your orange juice. INRA researchers (the French Agriculture Research Centre) have shown that if the amount of vitamins moderately drops during the first two months of conditioning in a glass packaging, it sharply drops and continue to decrease three, four months after the conditioning in the case of carton packaging.

So, what if you squeeze the oranges yourself? That is by far the best and only healthy option, but oranges are very acid and hard to metabolise for most people's stomach. It reinforces the acidosis of the body and will be hard to digest, especially when associated with a breakfast made of bread or cereals, as it is contradicting the gastric juices necessary to the digestion process. Also, orange juice is more acidic on your teeth than sodas or vinegar.

A simple test with a white chalk plunged in a glass of orange juice will be broken and soft after 10 minutes, a chalk plunged into a soda will show traces of erosion and colour, whereas it remains as it was in a glass of water. Therefore, if you drink sodas or juice, use a straw and do not brush your teeth before 30 minutes after absorption to avoid attacking your teeth enamel. Orange trees originated from India and China and were adapted to the climate of these countries. Today, most oranges are produced in Brazil, California, and Spain and are adapted to be eaten as a whole fruit between meals for people living under these Mediterranean or tropical climates. Living in New York, London, or Norway and drinking orange juice is more harmful than beneficial, leaving you with colder feet and hands and less energy—you should prefer lemon, parsley, broccoli, and kiwi as sources of vitamin C according to your body constitution. Parsley and broccoli juice? Why not being a trend setter!

Water

About 70 percent of our body is made of water. Yet, we often talk about nutrition without mentioning the importance of drinking pure and energised water. An adult usually drinks between 1.5 to 2.5 litres per day of water and absorbs 1.5 litres of water when taking a shower, so it is extremely important to choose the right water.

Tap water is the first source of water in our homes, but it is full of pesticides, nitrates, aluminium, heavy metals, chlorine, hormones (due to oral contraception that passes in the toilet pipes), and residues of medicine. Therefore drinking tap water not only should be avoided in industrialised countries but is unclean to consume in many developing countries.

Mineral waters are what most of us drink, usually from plastic bottles, which is in fact quite dangerous, especially in countries where temperatures are high. If you ever notice, it is written in small letters on the bottle, "do not put under light and heat" but by the time it reaches your local supermarket, your bottle of water has gone through quite a journey. The bottle PET (polyethylene terephthalate) might free antimony trioxide, which can severely damage the brain and liver. Therefore, always prefer glass bottles to plastic bottles when buying mineral waters.

However, according to various studies done in different European countries one out of five mineral waters is unsuitable for daily consumption. French waters, such as Evian or Vittel, are presented as chic and healthy waters abroad, whereas they are really only mediocre waters. Taking the local brand in a restaurant will cost you less for a product that has the same qualities.

Also, when buying a bottled mineral water, go for those with the smallest dry residue, if mentioned, or the smallest amount of calcium Ca+, sodium Na+, and fluoride F, as too high rates of these minerals are in fact fouling your body. The role of water is mainly to clean the body of its waste and not bring minerals that are usually too high for daily consumption. About 50 mg/litre maximum seems a reasonable figure for all these nutrients. Highly mineralised waters are, however, good for a punctual treatment given by your doctor, so process them with discernment.

Source water is usually much cheaper and much healthier than mineral waters, as they do not contain such high rates of minerals. Avoid purified or distilled water, which has undergone physical treatments to remove impurities and minerals that do not exist per se in nature. Instead of bringing hydration, purified or distilled water acidifies the body, leaches minerals and dehydrates the body. Because of its extreme purity, purified water absorbs carbon dioxide from the air, which makes it acidic and aggressive for our organism, not to mention that this water has completely lost its crystalline structure (no crystals are there to form a structure). Fereydoon Batmanghelidj, [18] an Iranian doctor, states in his bestselling book, Your Body's Many Cries for

---

[18] Batmanghelidj F. *Your body's many cries for water, the watercure* (2008).

Water that "The longer one drinks purified water, the more likely the development of mineral deficiencies and an acid state. Disease and early death is more likely to be seen with the long term drinking of purified water."

Many people in Europe and the United States have Brita-type pitchers to filter water at home. If Brita advertising claims to remove some chemicals, heavy metals such as lead, and the taste of chlorine, many studies raise doubts about it. This fails anyway to filter the medicine residue and chlorine, which is highly carcinogenic. And if the filter is not disinfected properly, bacteria multiply quickly and might be (in only one night) 20,000 times higher than what would be present in tap water.

Scientists and nutritionists talk a lot in recent years about inversed osmosed systems, which have been developed by NASA to recycle water used by astronauts. These systems are quite expensive (more than $1,000 USD in general, less for portable systems) but are useful to eliminate nitrates, pesticides, bacteria, limestone, mercury, lead, and other heavy metals to 95–98 percent and are worth investing in as water is the most important element of our nutrition and we often neglect it.

However, osmosed water is "dead water". It still lacks the energy that was lost in the water pipes and purification process. In nature, water runs down the river, flowing over stones and ground and is oxygenated naturally. Japanese researchers, like Professor Teruo Higa,[19] have worked on effective microorganism and EM ceramiques, which can energise the water and bring the millenary information back to water, thanks to special stones, ceramiques, and red mud. Laboratories have shown that these ceramiques allow water to find a coherent structure.

The vortex system is also an interesting revitalising system, which uses a swirling movement to bring back to water its kinetic movement and energise it.

The most important element in drinking a water of quality is the information given to the water. Waters in big cities are usually running in closed circuits carrying the same information, which is filled with stress, negative thoughts, and is reintroduced again and again in the pipes. In nature, the evaporation of water, which comes back in rain afterwards, allow the de-information, whereas it is not the case with water transported through pipes.

Scientists, such as Konstantin Korotkov, have shown that water can be informed positively or negatively and that it will affect the structure of water. Masuru Emoto[20] conducted an amazing study and photographed frozen crystals of water according to the information given to the water. Words such as "hate", "it's hopeless", "ugly," but also names such as "Hitler" make broken crystal shapes. Positive words such as

---

[19] Higa T. *Our future reborn: EM technology changes the world* (Sunmark Publishing, 2006).

[20] Emoto, A. *The miracle of water* (Atria, 2011).

"peace", "love", "you are beautiful", "adoration" said repeatedly to the water made beautiful crystal shapes, the most beautiful one being in fact two words "love and gratitude".

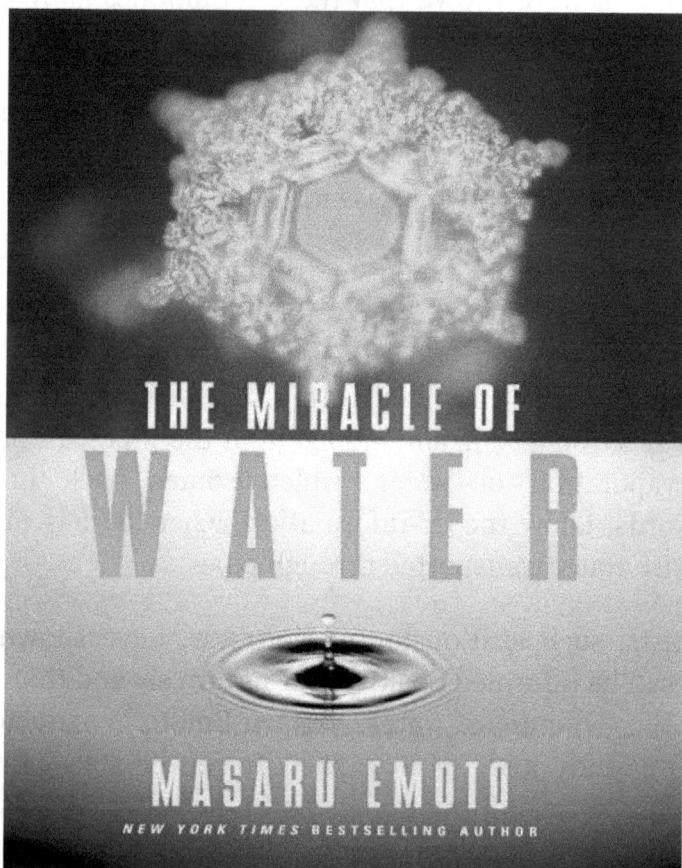

Love and gratitude crystal featured

You will learn in chapter 4 how to raise your own energy and raise the energy of water with simple techniques. Because whatever the water you drink, you can increase its vibrational level, and tap water that has been informed might sometimes have a higher vibration level than osmosed and energised water with the latest machines' technology. Also, as creatures made of 70 percent water, positive words and thoughts to ourselves have an amazing impact as we shall see in the next chapter with good food for our mind and spirit.

Fasting and detox

Fasting has been practised for centuries around the world and we are discovering again its benefits with the multiplication of fasting centres, fasting and walking holidays, etc. In Russia, for instance, fasting has been widely practised for decades. Thousands of pages of research and medical studies have been published during the Soviet era, but rarely translated into other languages, explaining why Western countries are lagging behind in terms of medical studies on fasting and fasting itself is not yet widespread.

Two of the oldest and most famous fasting clinics are the Buchinger clinics located in Uberlingen (Germany) and Marbella (Spain). I visited Marbella's five-star clinic standing out in a posh neighbourhood of the Andalusian recreational city. Here, people do not pay to eat tapas of fried calamari, chorizo, and other Spanish sausages. They come to fast in a high-tech clinic specialising in fasting therapies for more than 40 years.

The majority of the patients coming to the Buchinger clinic,[21] especially those from the Middle East, suffer from being overweight and primarily wish to lose weight and solve all their related health problems, such as diabetes 2, high rates

---

[21] Buchinger Clinic (in Uberlingen, Germany, and Marbella, Spain) is one of the many options offered for a fasting therapy.

of cholesterol, triglycerides, uric acid, hypertension, cardiac risks, etc. However, fasting is not a lifetime therapy that solves all the diseases or health problems. It is rather a lifestyle that every one of us should practise at least once a year to give our body and mind a break in the busy life that we are conducting all the year.

Losing weight is only one of the few side benefits of a fasting therapy but not the main one. Fasting is recommended in numerous diseases, as it gives the opportunity for the body to rest and find the necessary resources to operate the regeneration of cells and trigger the healing process.

A therapeutical fast will be recommended for the following diseases/ conditions: arthritis, chronic constipation, intestinal inflammation, migraines, headaches, menopause and premenstrual troubles, repetitive infections of the lungs, sinus problems, cystitis, allergies, acne, fertility issues, sclerosis, Parkinson's, Alzheimer's, fatigue, and fibromyalgia.

Fasting is not recommended for people with kidney or liver failure, anorexia, hyperthyroid, breastfeeding or pregnant women, or people treated for cancer during the chemotherapy phase. People with severe psychoses, addictions, duodenum and stomach ulcers, tumour diseases, and diabetes 1 can fast, but only under strict medical supervision.

Many organisations now offer fasting breaks of a week. From backpacking to five-star spa retreats, you have a wide range of possibilities.[22] Even if you are full of energy with vibrant health, it is always best to fast under medical supervision, especially for the first timers. Or use a detailed manual[23] about how to prepare, fast, and readapt your body after the fasting period. In all cases, the psychological and spiritual dimension is essential to get the maximum benefits of this break period.

In the three main monotheist religions, fasting is recommended and is even mandatory for Muslims during the month of Ramadan, where people partly fast for 28 to 29 days. Jesus fasted 40 days in the desert, so did Moses, and some Christians still follow a 40-day fast before Easter. Note that 40 days is usually the maximum physiological length that our body can stand.

In some Buddhist traditions, monks can fast for 72 days, but this happens only with an extreme spiritual preparation. Usually, there are some periods of 18- or 21-day fasts in many Asian traditions, such as reiki practitioners who practise this Japanese art of sacred energy, which heals themselves and others. The Buchinger clinic mentioned above and its founder, Otto Buchinger, recommended a period of 21 days, which has been reduced to 10 days to adapt to our modern lifestyle where most people cannot take 21 days for a fasting retreat.

---

22 For more information, visit www.haim.academy or your national fasting holiday organisations.

23 Wilhemi de Toledo F. *Therapeutic fasting, the Buchinger, Amplius method* (Thieme, 2011).

But before you undertake a real fast, I would recommend to fast one day per week to balance the excess of our modern diet, which is too rich and greasy. You can also do a monodiet or monomeal with rice, potatoes, or apples—a lot of options are available—and it allows your system to regenerate and rest. I noticed also that the prophet of Islam, Muhammad, recommended to fast one or two days per week, which is coherent with doctors' advice.

You can also skip a dinner meal for a week, especially after a party or trip where you have eaten more than usual to re-equilibrate your body, but it will be less efficient than a monomeal day.

Also, seasons are important. Spring and autumn are propitious to do a two- to three- week fast or detox, if you cannot get off work for such a long period. Plants, such as carrots, horseradish, artichokes, and green vegetables, such as spinach, help the organs eliminate the extra waste and detox the body. It is important to take care of the five main elimination doors of our system, which are the skin, the lungs, liver, intestines, and kidneys.

Therefore you should drink 1.5 to 2 litres per day of water and depurative herbal infusions (or take pills) such as desmodium adscendens, birch juice, sapwood, dandelion, according to the organ you want to detox. All the plants mentioned above support the cleansing of kidneys and liver, and can be used in a detox of 30 to 40 days during spring (March/April) and autumn (October/November).

It is better to check with a naturopath to be sure that your emunctory organs, your evacuation systems, work properly before doing a detox, as it might give you otherwise severe curative crises and side effects.

A global liver detox, called liver cleansing, is also recommended, at least once a year, more if your liver has been abused over the years. There are various methods to do it; one is the popular Andreas Moritz liver cleansing. It is easy to perform and takes seven days, from which one full day should preferably be spent at home, as you will evacuate toxins and gallstones.

Nevertheless, do not undertake a liver cleansing if you are currently under treatment or if you have a medical condition that might have a contraindication to do a liver detox. Also, only do a liver cleansing if your vital energy is high, as it might be counterproductive to do it if you are already lacking essential minerals and if your body is too exhausted to do a detox. If you have a doubt, you can best refer to your naturopath or your general practitioner for medical advice. Andreas Moritz book, *The amazing liver and gallbladder flush*[24] will give you a lot of information about the subject.

Fasting and detox periods are essential to our body, but they are also an occasion to align our body, mind, and spiritual needs and take this time to analyse what is beneficial to us in our lives and what changes we would like to make.

The vibration of the earth and the energy of food

The whole universe and all beings consist of energy and vibrate in harmony. In 1952, German scientist Winfried Otto Schumann discovered that there were electromagnetic

---

24 Moritz A. *The amazing liver and gallbladder flush* (Ener-chi Wellness Press, 2011).

standing waves in the atmosphere, within the cavity formed by the surface of the earth and the ionosphere, which are called the Schumann resonances.

His student, Herbert König, demonstrated a correlation between Schumann resonances and brain rhythms by measuring the oscillations of natural electromagnetic fields and performing electroencephalograms (measurement of the electrical activity of the brain along the scalp).

To put it succinctly, research studies on the Schumann resonances[25] show that the Earth has a vibrational level, vegetables have a vibrational level, animals and human beings have a vibrational level, which is almost the same under theoretical conditions.

One century before Schumann, a French trader and engineer, André Bovis, had the intuition that food elements had different energetic vibrations. He created a scale named after him to measure the vibrational level of foods.

His followers have since used the scale to measure a bit of everything, which is why the Bovis scale has been criticised. However, it remains a useful tool to measure the vibration of food, places, people, and so on.

Using a different basis of measurement, the Schumann resonances have proven scientifically that the earth has a

---

[25] Sentman DD. Schumann Resonances, Chapter 11. In Hans Volland (ed.). *Handbook of atmospheric electrodynamics,* Volume I (Boca Raton, Florida: CRC Press, 1995), 267.

constant vibration of 7.83 Hz, while geobiologists after Bovis have been using the notion of energetic levels empirically for a much longer period.

Food elements have different vibrations according to their mode of culture, intention, and information given to them. As for drugs and mobile phones, they have extremely low vibrational levels, as you should see in the box below.

The higher number, the better, and a good food energetic vibration should be close to the earth's vibration or at least above 8,000 Bovis units. Bear in mind that here we do not measure the food with calories but with its energy. Chinese doctors also use the energies of elements, using the concept of yin and yang to establish a diet for their patients.

Also, you might find different figures in older books, as the Earth's vibrational level is said to be constantly increasing and has undergone a drastic acceleration in the past 50 years, from 6,500 BU in the 1970s to 8,000 BU in the 1980–1990s up to 11,000 BU in 2015.

Vibration levels (in Bovis Unit, BU)

Cigarette 200–300
Mobile phone 1,600
Frozen pizza 3,700
Coffee 4,800
Big Mac sandwich 6,000
Veal meat from supermarket 5,800
Salmon 8,000
Local fresh fish brought to the village by fishermen 10,000
Germed seeds 10,600

Organic olive oil made in family garden 10,000
Organic oil bought in supermarket 8,500
Sunflower oil, retailer brand 8,500

Lemon 7,000
Organic lemon 8,500
Tomato (supermarket) 7,300
Organic tomato 8,500
Organic tomato from family garden 9,500
Organic tomato from family garden after one minute informing with
    light, love and ask God to bless the food 12,500

Vegetable soup 9,000
Same vegetable soup left in the fridge for one day 7,000
Frozen vegetables bought in supermarket 5,900

Tap water 8,000
Mineral water 9,500
Source water 10,000

Desinformed water* 10,500
Informed tap water with Peace and Love 11,500
Informed source water with Peace and Love 13,000

* The water has been left for two hours in a glass bottle under the sun.

The way to interpret these measurements is quite simple: some activities and some food give you energy, while other things deplete your energy. If the earth vibration is now around 11,000 BU, it means that a healthy person vibrates at

11,000. If this person has a healthy lifestyle and spiritual activity, she will quickly raise to 13,000 or 15,000 or 18,000 BU. Some spiritual leaders are higher than 50,000 BU, such as Pope Francis or the Dalai Lama.

If the person is tired, depressed or ill, the vibration will decrease below 11,000. To each illness, there is also a corresponding vibrational level. And most of the industrial food we eat has the vibration of cancer or HIV (as illnesses also have a given vibration), which means that this food is not really energetic.

To increase our energy and vibrational level, our thoughts, meditative activities, and prayers are important, but food is the first source of our daily energy, so it is important to buy food that has a good energy level. By eating organic food, you enjoy food with a higher energy level nurturing you and giving you strength. Also, when you eat something that is raw and alive, you find more energy in it.

Meat or fish is from a dead animal. Although it contains proteins and the eight essential amino acids, its energetic level is much lower than germed seeds, for instance, which contain proteins. Antibiotics, vaccinations, conditions of farming, and pollutions of the oceans also explain why the energetic level of the animals we eat is usually low.

But also, information is an important parameter, which can influence the energetic level of the food. When a small fisherman sells the catch of the day, it has most probably less stress and negative energies than fish processed by big companies looking for maximal profit, where the fish has been loaded and deloaded so many times, without mentioning the conditions of fishing and employment of the workers.

Cigarettes, drugs, alcohol, and industrial food all deplete our energy. Electromagnetic fields are also disturbing our vital energy. This also affects the animals and the environments we live in without us knowing exactly what are the consequences. It will take a few years before there are impact studies about their effect on our health.

Eat at peace!

Eating in front of an action or horror movie is just so bad for your body! Eating requires our body to be focussed on the nutrients it ingests and enjoy the food it takes in. Therefore, always try to eat in a peaceful and quiet environment, without a TV screen on, as you will spare yourself a lot of electromagnetic fields. Also bad news, stressful images, and unuseful activity for your eyes and brain during this period will affect you. I often noticed that when I used to eat at work with colleagues talking about problems not only did I have a strong stomach pain after eating but also I felt more hungry after I had food than before, which is what you feel also when you eat in fast-food. I am sure you have experienced such situations already, so you know what I am talking about.

In Indian medicine, Ayurveda, people are made of one dominant dosha, or type, and a huge emphasis is put on the eating environment, which should be peaceful and silent, especially for people of the kapha, earth people. If you have noticed, monks of Christian monasteries or Buddhists eat in silence. In many Asian cultures, speaking too much or having a business lunch is considered to harm your body and spoil the food, which should be respected and eaten in silence.

Therefore, try to eat slowly, in a positive environment, and if you are eating alone and feel emptiness, you can listen to calm and relaxing music—lounge, rock, and techno music stresses your body. Restaurant chains use loud rhythmic music to "awaken and arouse your senses," that is, to say, make their customers eat more food.

Exercise!

Doing regular exercise is actually part of a healthy diet. Walking after a meal will not only help the digestion process but also bring oxygen to your muscles and brain. If you are not used to walking, you should start with 10 minutes at least four times a week. It can be only a walk around your house, but you might prefer to go to the beach if you live near the sea or in a park if you live in the city centre. Walking near trees helps you get rid of your own used energies and renew your energy as we shall see in chapter 4.

Your ultimate goal should be to walk 40 minutes, three times a week or 1 hour and 15 minutes twice a week. If you practise other sports, this is excellent and you should continue doing it, but walking should be incorporated into your program. Remember, always adapt your physical activities to your abilities. Many doctors recommend swimming, as it is good for your muscles and the skeleton but, it should be done in natural water (see, ocean, lakes, and rivers) as swimming pools are full of chloride, which can provoke cancer in the long run, not to mention various venereal diseases.

Stretching, Pilates, and other fitness activities are also excellent to increase your energy flow, elasticity, and breathing abilities, but choose carefully the type of practise you wish to do and adapt it to your physical condition. Exercising is also a fantastic food for your mind, as it frees serotonin, the happiness hormone, and oxytocin, the hormone that manages pleasure and balance. Oxytocin is also commonly called the sex hormone, as it is liberated during pleasant intercourse.

Chapter 2

Food for My Mind and Spirit

We are doing a lot of effort to build our image and reflect a positive opinion of ourselves. We spend a lot of time and money to buy creams to hydrate our skin, to reduce wrinkles; we invest in organic foods, special diets; we buy expensive perfumes and apply fancy make-up to cover-up imperfections so as to appear healthy and in good shape . . . but what do we do to take care of our mind and our spirit? Can you imagine if we could just go to Galeries Lafayette (the fancy retail shop in Paris) and find counters of soul-regenerating creams, dark-stain removers, energy injections . . . oh, and maybe a bit further around the Chanel stand a wonderful brand called "Renouveau," which applies a mask to your face to decongest negative thoughts, remove them gently with a hot wet towel, and apply an orange flower regenerating cream that renews your cells and allows a brand new thinking? Wouldn't it be fantastic?

Unfortunately, there is no fast beauty track for our mind. It requires work from our side. And maybe we do not put effort into it because we think it is not as obvious as our physical body. But as we know, already our body language shows something of ourselves—confidence, sincerity, and success, or shyness, discomfort, and dishonesty. Why is this so? Because our brain, our thoughts, directly reflect on our physical body. We can artificially adopt postures and attitudes that will help us look as we want during a date or job interview, but the truth is that our first impression does not last.

We cannot lie about our inner state for long because we communicate a kind of energy that is either positive or negative. Why do we immediately like or dislike someone? Why do some people actually do nothing wrong but you just feel uncomfortable being with them? We emit a vibration and transmit an energy that resonates with what is around us, sometimes the frequency will be adequate to our own vibration, sometimes it will just conflict. And we can notice that the more we adopt a positive attitude, the more we will attract people like ourselves, and the more we are depressed, the more we will attract negative or depressed people to us, this can be called the attraction law or the resonance law.

We are the master of our mind. Our mind is powerful and our thoughts influence the world around us. Positive thoughts have the power not only to keep us healthy but also to communicate positive energy, which will be given back to us. Have you ever noticed that when you are in a queue at the supermarket and you start grunting, having in your mind all kinds of bird names for the cashier, it usually ends up in a fight even before you speak a word? On the contrary, have you been able during a fight with your boss, or when witnessing a violent scene, to send peace and love to the protagonists and see things resolved quickly? This is exactly what our thoughts can do.

Masaru Emoto,[26] who passed away in 2014, extensively studied the influence of words and thoughts on crystals of water. By freezing drops of water that he later examined with a microscope and by informing them with various words, such as love, joy, dislike, or hopeless, or names of people, such as Hitler or Mother Teresa, crystals had totally different shapes! They were either harmonious and beautiful, or broken and disrupted. My favourite, which was also Emoto's, looks like a snow star. This is the "love and gratitude" crystal . . . once you see it, you will remember it for the rest of your life. The earth and our bodies are made of up to 70 percent water, which means that the information we gives ourselves either brings harmony to our bodies or distress and illnesses.

Also, Emoto conducted an experiment with rice. He left three pots of cooked rice in a table and did the following experiment. To one of them, he sent love every morning and wrote "love" on the pot. The second one was left ignored. The third one was informed with negative thoughts with the word "you fool" written on the pot. Many people have tried the same experiment at home with the same compelling results.

After three weeks, the first pot of rice was still perfectly white, while the second one had a lot of dark spots and mould in it, and the third one was really black and rotten. If rice reacts so much to different information and thoughts, imagine how we humans are influenced by the thoughts that people send us and the thoughts that we give to ourselves!

---

26 Emoto, A. *The miracle of water* (Atria, 2011).

We might not change at first what others think about us, but we can definitely change what we think about ourselves!

Healthy habits

Having positive thoughts requires work exactly like an athlete trains every day in order to be fit. As we change our thoughts, we will see our life changing: positive people will come around us, we will experience fewer negative events during our day and we will be happier.

Negative thoughts do not only affect our brains, but they also affect our physical bodies because we are made of energy and information. Emotional shocks, conflicts penetrate our energetic bodies located around our physical body, and if they are too strong, they will reach the physical body, causing various disorders and illnesses.

This is why creating healthy mind habits is important and coordinates your efforts towards a healthy lifestyle. Aristotle said, "We are what we do repeatedly". Excellency is not an action it is a habit". And to create this habit you will need to stretch yourself and persistently pursue practicing new habits for about a month, or 21[27] days as mentioned by researcher William James. The number 21 is important: the prophet Daniel fasted 21 days as do Christians doing Daniel fasting, Buddhists fast 21 days, Buchinger clinics advise a 21-day fast to clean the body and mind, reiki has to be practised

---

[27] James W. *Writings 1878–1899: Psychology, talks to teachers and students* (Library of America, 1992).

for 21 days on oneself before being used as a healing method for others etc.

Being a happy person is achievable by every person who decides it and consistently applies a daily routine in her life, which will ensure present and future happiness.

Exactly like becoming healthy or having a nice body shape requires constant exercise, having a healthy mind and spirit requires avoiding things that keep us unhealthy and practise instead habits that will lead us to be balanced. Being happy is not taught at school, unless you went to Harvard University and followed Tal Ben-Shahar[28] and his class on happiness. Therefore, you will need to establish a routine of your own. I humbly hope to give you keys here to do so.

---

[28] Ben-Sharar T. Happier: *Learn the secret to daily joy and lasting fulfillment* (McGraw-Hill, 2007).

Organise your life for success

What do successful people do? Is this just mere luck or inherited from their family? I don't believe so. Success and happiness is something you reach and live by having a daily routine that transforms you and makes you become the person you will be tomorrow. Tom Corley* studied for five years the habits of 233 rich people and 128 people living in poverty and measured some key elements which bring success.

- 88% of the rich read 30 minutes per day for their education versus 2% of the poor.
- 86% of the rich continue to learn and get education versus 5% of the poor.
- 67% of wealthiest watch one hour less of TV every day versus 23% of the poor.
- 6% of the wealthy watch TV reality shows versus 78% of the poor.
- 84% believe good habits create opportunity luck versus 4% of the poor.
- 76% of the rich exercise at least four times per week versus 33% of the poor.
- 67% of the wealthy write their dreams versus 11% of the poor.
- 70% of wealthy parents make their children volunteer 10 hours or more per month versus 3% of the poor.

* Corley, Tom, *Rich Habits—the daily success habits of wealthy individuals* Langdon Street Press, 2010).

Get rid of negative thoughts

What we think today determines who we will be in the future. And what we think today will influence our mental state and our global health. Therefore, it is important to be firm and violent with our negative thoughts. You can read and say the following sentence out loud now: THERE IS NO SPACE FOR ANY NEGATIVE THOUGHTS IN MY MIND NOW. Once again read out loud this sentence: THERE IS NO SPACE FOR MY NEGATIVE THOUGHTS (IN MY MIND) NOW. Consistently repeating this sentence each time a bad thought occurs, each time you feel depressed, angry, sad, or stupid is essential to the shifting process. I started by saying this sentence 30 times a day. I now have to say it two or three times a day. I realised that I used to feed my brain with negative thoughts all day long, which was even encouraged and emphasised by studying in the most competitive universities of the country, by working as a journalist in a newsroom where pressure is constant, by hearing from my childhood that it is not enough, that I have to do more, etc. . . . We all have our little negative push buttons around us and our own story. It does not matter what your story is, just focusing on noticing and rebuking each negative thought as it occurs will already be a big step towards achieving a positive mindset.

Speak life to yourself

Do you see how fat you are? How stupid you look? How big your nose is? Why do you always do that? No one will ever like you. From our childhood we heard negative comments from our teachers, sometimes our parents, some people made fun of us . . . all this leaves stains in us and prevents us from being the great person that we are meant to be . . . and, most often, these comments mentioned above are made by ourselves . . . we often are our biggest enemy!

One of the big soap companies[29] made an experiment by filming women in front of the mirror asking them to say out loud what they were saying to themselves in their mind . . . then, they would go to a group session with the other women

---

29 Dove by Nivea, not to mention it.

participating in the experience and at some point, one of the ladies would say the same comment to the author of this ugly thought . . . they were totally shocked and in awe at how much violence they gave to themselves.

What we speak to ourselves is therefore important. One verse of the Bible mentions "the power of tongue is life and death" (Proverbs 18:21), and it is in the end literally true. If I tell myself every day that I will die soon, that I am going to have cancer, that I will never succeed, etc., it is quite probable that it will occur like a self-fulfilling prophecy.

On the contrary, if I wake up every morning, and I automatically say, whatever the weather, taste of the coffee, outside temperature, pressure of the water in the shower, "this is a beautiful day, I am going to enjoy it", or "I am a great person and I am healthy, successful, and beautiful", I promise you that in six to eight weeks you will not be the same person anymore and that everyone around you will notice it!

If you have children, always remember that one sentence only can change their destiny, and I really mean their entire life. My younger sister of seven years, Manon, was a disappointing pupil at elementary school. Not only was she 40 percent deaf, she did not study properly nor did she put much effort in it. Until one day when she won the city competition for young violin players. My mother commented and said "even your sister never succeeded to do that"! From that day, not only she became the best pupil of her class, and it lasted until high school where she passed her diploma with the highest grades, but she also recovered her full hearing capacity in about three months.

Maybe her ears did not want to hear any more negative comments and receive this violence, unconsciously. Just one sentence can change the destiny of a child! And repeated comparisons between children can just condemn some of them to be the lame duck of the family when there is absolutely nothing wrong with them but with the projection of their parents. The power of tongue is life and death, remember it!

Organising a positive and energetic environment for ourselves

We usually spend half our life at home, sometimes even more for self-employed people or housewives. Establishing a positive environment at home where you can feel energy flowing in is important. Feng-shui art is a powerful tool to place furniture and decorations in a way that will make you feel comfortable and relaxed. It needs many books and long hours to describe all its possibilities but as a first step, removing mirrors from your bedroom, especially facing the bed or on the ceiling will allow you to sleep better. You can also move your bed 40 to 50 cm from the wall, as walls usually carry a waveform aggregating unclean energies—especially if you do not live in a flat or house where you are the first occupant.

Using different colours to decorate the room according to the effect desired also helps to harmonise the place. For instance, red or orange are great colours to stimulate energy and grounding and can be applied on kitchen walls or in the living room. Light blue or purple will favour calm, meditation, intuition, and can be applied in an office or your bedroom. But above all, computers, Wi-Fi, mobile phones, and TV sets are the first devices to switch off at night as they emit strong electromagnetic waves even on a sleep position.

Moreover, what you use as decorations is important as it is filled with vibrations and history. Try to remove all unnecessary decorations, especially presents and antiques from your grandparents, collections of puppets, vases, etc. . . . always be wary of the furniture you buy in second-hand shops as it carries the energy of the people who had it in their home.

Some would argue that buying new furniture made in developing countries, such as China where workers work in difficult conditions often underpaid and undernourished, carries anger, fear, or hate energies. In any case, I would recommend you to wash all your furniture with sea water or salt and water with a sponge to make the energies new and neutral. If it is antique furniture, you can use beeswax and visualise that this furniture is now cleaned.

Also, as a health measure, all furniture made of pressed wood and glue (typically IKEA and all main brands) should remain in a room with its windows open or on a balcony for 15 days, the time for the solvent to evaporate. There is nothing worse than to buy a new wardrobe and put it immediately in a child's bedroom, as his or her lungs and breathing organs are more sensitive than adults, and they will breathe solvent contained in the glue.

I also know many people who hang pictures of ancestors and dead beloved ones in the living room. I would advise to remove them, as it carries the energy of these people and makes you stay in the past instead of going forward. It is to be noted that in China people believe that pictures of dead people are to be removed, as it is believed that they bring negative spirits or energy.

Also, placing posters of singers, athletes, statues of saints, Venetian masks, and African masks is not neutral and brings a special energy to the place, not to say negative in many cases. The Quai Branly museum in Paris exposes thousands of African masks and primitive civilisation objects. I noticed that most of the energy therapists, pastors, Feng-shui practitioners, or spiritual people all told me they felt bad in this particular museum and had the impression that some kind of spirits were around the place . . . . pure imagination or exaggeration for some, reality of a spiritual world that is totally denied in the West, part of the daily life of African, Asian, or South American civilisations, I always prefer to apply the precautionary principle and would advise not to have these objects at home.

Posters with war images or negative quotations are to be removed, as again it is before your eyes every day and works in your subconscious and spirit negatively. In any case, all objects that you feel are filled with unknown or negative energies should be thrown away. I was given two vases by my grandmother. They were designed with steel shell casings during World War II by soldiers she had hidden in her home. They were beautiful and it was a masterpiece of history, but I removed them and sold them to a collector (as they were carrying the energies of suffering, fear, violence, etc.).

Symbols and stones can be helpful, but they often stimulate good energies or bad energies. For instance, the triskele sign helps raise the energy of a place, but it stimulates everything that is present in the room, the good and the bad . . . therefore, it can awaken bad memories, sadness, and anger, without you realising it. On the contrary the Star of David, which recalls the spider web prophet David hid behind as he was purchased by soldiers of Saul, and later used also by prophet Muhammad in the Athal grotto to hide from his pursuers, would protect against the negative radiation of electromagnetic fields. Alternative healers suggest placing a six-branch star on the electrical meter, or in your pocket to protect you and your home. Yoga practitioners use a star to stimulate chakras of the heart. And many Jews nowadays still wear a golden Star of David as a community symbol and also as a protection symbol.

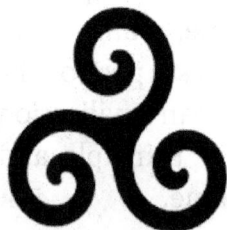

Triskele

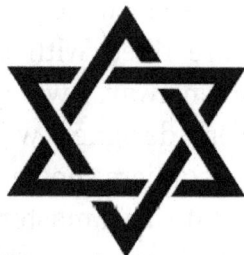

Star of David

In the end, the lighter your home decoration will be, the better your mind and spirit will feel. Fortunately, new design styles are going into the direction of minimalism! Scandinavian design, which embodies this minimalism with natural woods, light colours, and design, brings peace and space to the place.

Choose your clothes

Clothes are on our skin all day and night long. It is therefore important to be aware of what we are wearing. This is for physical reasons, but also for spiritual reasons as colours, designs, and inscriptions transfer.

Natural materials, such as cotton, wool, linen, and silk, should be preferred whenever possible. Again, it depends on the condition of its production. Greenpeace releases an annual index of environmentally toxic clothes, which can be helpful in choosing clothes to buy, but usually anything cheap, produced by mainstream brands in developing countries is not the guarantee of healthy, quality clothing. Also, synthetic clothing can provoke strong incompatibility to the person wearing it who will have muscle pain, reduced movement abilities, headaches, psoriasis, etc.

A French doctor, Gérard Dieuzaide, extensively studied the subject and, for him, almost all materials, especially synthetic cloth, can be unsuitable, the problem being that it is personal to each and every one of us. My neighbour can feel well in a viscose T-shirt, while I will have a strong disturbance wearing it. The same applies to jewellery and glasses, which can be incompatible for some people.

In the 1960s, a doctor from Nice, France, Jean-Pierre Maschi, published a tendentious comparative study on sclerosis rate between Nordic countries and Maghreb. He found that in countries such as Morocco, where people mainly wore cotton and wool clothes with leather sandals, the baboosh, sclerosis was almost nonexistent at the time. Whereas in Nordic countries, where people wore synthetic materials and boots with gum below to isolate from the cold, sclerosis rates were very high. His hypothesis was that non-natural material and shoes, which isolate our feet from the ground, were the reason for the development of that illness. Whatever the issues he had with the doctors' council in France, first radiated then rehabilitated in his job, it is worth paying attention to our clothing material and protect our health.

But it is also essential to pay attention to the design and inscriptions written as it has a power, like saying words out loud. It gets even recorded in our energetic body located around us, transmitting information to our body. Wearing a T-shirt where it is written for instance " I am a bitch", "I am possessed by the devil, don't come near", or where dead skulls are painted, weapons, and negative images definitely have a negative impact on our mood consciously, but also on the unconscious and spiritual level for our energy bodies and our spirit. Words and images are power! Do not forget it.

Colours that you wear also have the same impact as the walls of your home. If you choose to wear plain black clothes, be aware that black absorbs energies while white reflects it. Black is a colour that absorbs energy, good or bad. Priests wear black as if they were collecting people's negative energies during their confession of sins. White reflects energy, which is why spiritual leaders wear it, as it feeds their energy around.

Have you noticed that doctors and health practitioners wear white uniforms, which reflects energy, or green uniforms, which is the heart chakra colour and the healing colour? Hospitals and pharmacies have green signs and walls, for instance. People who wear black clothes, such as Gulf women who wear long abaya gowns, should put a coloured ribbon (preferably red, orange, or yellow) into their underwear, or wear coloured underwear and clothes to maintain a good vibratory level.

Paying attention to our environment and ourselves is as important as buying all the best food we can afford. Carefully choosing clothes, enjoying a home filled with peace and harmony in its design are also mind foods that will help our bodies to be healthy and light. You might not have thousands of dollars to change your home and your wardrobe but paying attention and making affordable changes (you can even make some money by selling unnecessary decorations and equipment) will greatly improve your well-being.

Food for our mind in a technological world

Food for our mind is as important as the solid food or even more so, because we do not live on bread and water alone, but we are creatures with a mind, a conscious that helps us think and do things thoughtfully. I believe today that most of the food we feed to our minds comes from the TV, the videos from the Internet, and social media. In the past 20 years, our dependency on technological devices has completely changed our time schedule, our family life, our couple life, and our work life.

Technology has definitely impacted the way we think and the way we live, not to mention that it might impact the way we die with the electromagnetic waves projected to our bodies for which we do not have reliable studies to evaluate its harm. There are a lot of wonderful things on TV, on the Internet, and on social media. My aim here is not to put forward an extreme point of view but to give you keys that will help you make your choices for a healthy lifestyle.

TV, an unnecessary food for my mind

More than 90 percent of people have a TV set in the Western countries (99 percent in the United States, but "only" 93 percent in Finland) and Americans spend on average 6 hours 47 minutes per day in front of their TV, which means that if you are like me, one of the remaining 1 to 5 percent of people who do not have a TV at home, you are rather a kind of alien of the twenty-first century.

Surprisingly, I have been a huge TV consumer at work. I have worked for seven years as a journalist for international 24/7 news channels, such as CNN, BBC, and France 24. So, you might wonder why I do not have a TV at home. Because I worked for too long in the news industry, I know the impact of TV programs on our physical health and mental health dealing with negative information all day long. At the last radio broadcast station I worked for, among 70 journalists, 30 of them were on heavy medication to treat depression and anxiety, so many people aged less than 35 had multiple bone and muscle problems . . .

I, myself, was unable to move my arm and neck for three months due to the pressure, content, and atmosphere at work. People working for the media usually work in a frustrating and pressuring environment, not to mention that the shifting working patterns have consequences on their mental health, which is reflected in the content produced. Do you want to watch content made by people who are hit by negativity and mental issues? Information and energy are transmitted by vibrations and waves . . . although it is only in your TV, it still comes to you at home.

When you get negative energies or produce negative thoughts, it is like a cloud over your head. You meet other people who also have a cloud of negativity over their heads and these clouds aggregate together and get bigger. Imagine these negative clouds meet a positive person, it will probably contaminate him/her unless the person is strong enough in which case it will not stay over his/her energetic body and the cloud will look for someone else, but it is not the most likely scenario. When you get used to a cloud of negativity over your head, you do not notice anymore that it is negative ... the more you watch TV, the more you get used to violence or bad news . . . but if you stop watching it for several months, you might be shocked that you barely tolerate pictures and stories that were your daily food only a few months before.

In the end, are TV, news, and movies really a good thing for our physical, mental, and spiritual health? And I don't mean here to start a debate about the content of the news we watch, which often provoke fear, anxiety, and might sometimes (or often . . .) be biased by various interests.

Aletha Huston[30] at the University of Texas (USA), studied 100 preschool children watching cartoons. Some children on the panel watched cartoons with violence, others without. Her report states that "children who watch violent shows, even funny cartoons, were more likely to hit at their playmates, argue, disobey class rules, leave tasks unfinished and were less willing to wait". The occurrence of guns on our TV screens increased by 85 percent between 1998 and 2002

---

30 Huston AC. *Fair child, big world, small screen. The role of TV in the American society* (University of Nebraska Press, 1992).

(no data available 10 years later), which means our brain records more and more violent events even passively.

For centuries and millenaries, men were observing violence only when it was before their eyes, and although witnessing a murder or torture could happen, it was less likely to be observed so many times a day. You might say, "It is only a movie, it is only TV" but the brain and cells record this violence despite a rational analysis that says it is not real.

This violence really affects our body and also our mind and spirit. An average child in the United States watches 12,000 violent acts on TV (murder, assault . . .) annually, which means an average of 20 acts per hour[31]! And I do not think results might be very different in other countries as trends and programs are more or less the same around the world. We are far from even the fiercest warriors of Genghis Khan at his time!

Reading develops one's imagination, while cooking, sewing, gardening, and drawing keeps us grounded. TV is a passive activity, which fills the brain instead of giving some free space to think. TV emits strong electromagnetic fields even on the sleep position. So you should always switch it off totally and put it away from your bedroom as it still emits small electromagnetic fields and watching the screen before sleeping gives excitement to the brain and neurotransmitters.

---

[31] Gerbner G. and Signorelli N. *Violence and terror in the mass media* (New York: Greenwood Press, 1988).

For those using computers, installing an application that turns your screen yellowish at night will reduce the inconvenience of the blue light of the screen for your eyes, or using special glasses[32] will also help, but it is best to avoid using smartphones, tablets, computers, and TVs before sleeping. In addition, you should always watch your TV at a distance of five times the diagonal width of the screen to avoid exposure to its electromagnetic fields . . . but, by now, you have already rushed to a second-hand sales website to sell your TV or throw it away in your garbage . . . Am I right?

If not, try to pay attention to the time you spend in front of the TV and for which kind of program. And if you are like the 66 percent of Americans who eat in front of the TV set,[33] I would encourage you to reread the section about food and the importance of eating at peace and in a calm environment. Not everyone has to eat in silence, like Buddhist or Christian monks around the world, but lunch and dinner might be the perfect time to exchange with your spouse or children or listen to relaxing music if you live alone.

Mobile phones, social media, do we need a social detox?

More than 860 million mobile phones and 940 million smartphones were sold in the world in 2014. There are 93 mobile phones per 100 inhabitants worldwide (2013) while

---

32 Gunnar glasses, not to mention them.

33 Three screen report—A quarterly analysis from Nielsen's Anywhere Anytime Media Measurement initiative (A2/M2) (2nd quarter 2009).

there was only 0.6 mobile per 100 inhabitants in the world, for instance, in 1993.[34] Facebook claims 1.44 billion users worldwide—77 percent of American teens aged 12 to 17 use Facebook, and 47 percent of the 18–34 year olds use social media or texting during meals.[35] About 42 percent of French people sleep with their mobile phone on next to their bed, 73 percent of students and teenagers [36] and 51 percent of executives read and reply to emails in their bed . . . the trend to read emails, look at social media feed, and text in the bedroom is so widespread that a famous company making condoms[37] has even launched a global campaign, certainly after noticing a decline in sales, to encourage people to switch off their mobile phones in order to have more intimacy with their partner!

On a physical level, mobile phones emit a strong electromagnetic field, so does your wireless connection. Therefore, you should switch them off at night (or set your mobile phone on the airplane mode). There are a lot of devices on the market to reduce their impact on our health with various efficiencies. Some of these devices even allow reversing the negative waves (vertically polarised waves) into positive vibrations for the body (dextrorotatory turns). You

---

[34] ARTE Program, Le dessous des cartes (below the maps). (2015).

[35] Pan J. Tweets at the tables? More of us mix social media and food.

[36] Study by the National Institute of Sleep INSV / MGEN. Sommeil et environnement (sleep and environment). (2013).

[37] Durex.

can put a sticker on your phone or a special plate on your electrical meter or use a mattress that uses the scalar waves technology, which will help you recharge your batteries and lower the effects of the electromagnetic fields on your body. I tried it and I definitely felt like sleeping in heaven! This said, the digital age not only affects us physically but also mentally and energetically, as this intense over-communication paradoxically develops loneliness and dependency syndromes. An American study reported that people were reporting less face-to-face time with their family—from 8 percent in 2000 to 34 percent 2011. Most people (58 percent of adult smartphone users and 68 percent of young adults) do not go one hour without checking their emails or Facebook notifications, making it hard for them to concentrate on a task or a special moment . . . on average, we check our mobile phone 150 times per day![38]

When was the last time you had coffee with a friend and none of you answered a call or checked something on your mobile phone? Mobile phones so much changed our lives that several detox centres[39] have opened recently to help mobile phone addicts to disconnect. During the week these centres help you to reconnect with yourself, to communicate with others, and to find the right balance among digital activities and real life. Addiction and mobile phone compulsive use even have created new psychological issues such as the Fear of Missing Out (FOMO) or the phantom

---

[38] Ahonen T. Main trends in the telecommunications market.
     Presentation at MoMo mobile conference, Kiev, Ukraine. (2011).

[39] See Shambhalaranch.com.

vibration syndrome—a perceived vibration from a cell phone that is not vibrating. You can check and tick the boxes of our addiction survey here . . . if you ticked more than five sentences you should definitely find some time to establish a digital detox!

CROSS EVERY TIME YOU:

- ☐ Feel a phantom vibration.
- ☐ Reach for your phone.
- ☐ Have the urge to look something up.
- ☐ Checking your email.
- ☐ Want to call someone to say hi.
- ☐ Feel like posting an update or checking in.
- ☐ Want to take a picture or selfie.
- ☐ Look for your phone.
- ☐ Experience FOMO (fear of missing out).

I started my digital detox two years ago, when I noticed that even if I had quit my work as a journalist, I was compulsively checking news from morning to evening and sometimes when I was waking up at night, checking Twitter, Facebook at least once per hour and suffering from neck and shoulder pain due to my compulsive chatting on the phone. I started my digital detox by deliberately leaving my mobile phone one hour per week at home, which became one day per week! A digital Shabbat makes you so relaxed! And closing your Facebook account will save you so much time! I did not lose any job opportunity, or any real friends, despite all my prejudices that being disconnected might be really bad for my social life. And let's face it, our time spent for professional reasons on social media does not represent more than 10 percent of it . . . so let's be honest and enjoy disconnection for a bit!

Facebook transforms our life in a way that we do not live for ourselves anymore but for others who will watch our profile feed. Years ago we were taking pictures for ourselves or our close family, which we could make sit on a sofa to watch our latest holiday pictures. Nowadays, we often think about what kind of picture we could put on Facebook to document our best moments. After I closed my Facebook account, I sometimes caught myself thinking, "I wish I had Facebook to post this beautiful picture" showing the impact that social media has on our daily life.

I have a friend who is a public speaker and she admitted finding herself taking twenty times the same picture of her preparing for a lecture at her desk, changing the position of books she places first on her desk wondering which ones will look better on the picture . . . we all recall these experiences when we tried to show the best of ourselves. Our world is more and more competitive. And it has become a competition to show who has the best pictures on Facebook, whom we are having dinner with, the trendy event we attend . . . which is in the end, only postpones the illusion to live a fulfilling life when it is only an illusion or delusion intended for others.

Facebook is responsible for 20 percent of the divorces in the United States, and I am sure it might be the case in many other countries around the world. It even makes people stay more in their past and develop biased relationships. I had so many friends checking the Facebook page of their former boyfriend to see what "he was up to"; other friends have broken up with their partner as he/she did not mention on his Facebook that he/she is "in a relationship", or jealous and nasty competitors sometimes put up old pictures where they stand with the man/woman they love . . . bringing all kinds of fights, frustrations, and angers spurred by a virtual world, stealing here their real life and happiness.

For those who have children, it is even more important to watch closely their use of technology as their brains and eyes are sensitive to screens, electromagnetic fields, and information they see. Did you know that Apple's Steve Jobs did not allow his kids to use a tablet or an iPhone? Once asked during an interview about what did his children think about iPad, he replied: "they do not have any".[40]

Did you know that most Silicon Valley tycoons and social media CEOs (to quote Twitter's Evan Williams) do not let their children use a mobile phone before they are 14 years old and restrict their access to social media? Most of these top-end employees of high-tech companies register their kids in private schools where technology is not used at all. Waldorf schools in California and across the United States are some of these schools where kids learn knitting, gardening, and cooking but do to know how to do a Google search before they are 14 years old. As American teenagers (and others around the world) now spend 7 hours, 30

---

[40] Bilton N. Steve Jobs was a low-tech parent. *New York Times* (10.09.2014).

minutes in front of a screen every day,[41] it is crucial to review our position towards technology and use it in a healthy and smart way.

Music, a message to the soul

"Give me control over he who shapes the music of a nation, and I care not who makes the laws," said Napoleon. Music is not only notes and rhythm being played in the background. It is a direct message to our soul. Many studies have been conducted to know which kind of music allows retailers to sell more, to make people stay longer in a place, relax more, study more, etc. What is definitely obvious is that exactly like good food, good thoughts, and good decorations brings positive energy to us, good music allows our spirit to connect with its higher self.

Some music genres on the contrary induce violent behaviours, depressions, and negative thoughts. Rap music with a high content of violent speeches and explicit video clips favour violent attitudes and delay academic performance. [42] It leads its listeners to have a wider acceptance of violence, especially against women. It is now public knowledge that many rap singers or other pop singers had to go through blood deals to get to sign a contract with big labels. Trading off close friends or family in various ways

---

[41] Broadcaster Audience Research Board. (2011).

[42] Johnson JD, Jackson LA, and Gatto, L. Violent attitudes and different academic aspirations: Deleterious effects of exposure to rap music. *Basic and applied social psychology* 16, 1–2, (1995): 27–41.

to get a chance to get money and success is something that is not mentioned in mass media but does exist. It put into question the "energy" of people producing music. The music industry is a keystone of mind shaping and mind shifting in our societies, because it allows reaching the furthest and deepest part of our mind and soul.

Jazz music is also an interesting music style for sociologists and psychologists. It is associated with people who have high self-esteem, creative and outgoing people,[43] high income, but customer behaviour analysis, for instance, shows that when jazz is played in a restaurant, people leave the place in less than one hour, compared to lounge, pop, or classical music where people stay much longer. But jazz is the music that makes customers at a restaurant spend the most money. What better option for a restaurant to make your customers leave the premises quickly and spend a lot of money?

Jazz is also considered to be a spiritual music designed to relax the mind, but studies shows that on the contrary, that is not the case at all. A study conducted on horses show that jazz music and rock music are the music styles that make the horses display the more stressful behaviours and disturbed eating patterns, with jazz being the most aversive of all kinds of music on horses.[44]

---

[43] North AC and Hargreaves DJ. *The social and applied psychology of music* (Oxford: Oxford University Press, 2008).

[44] Carter C and Greening L. Auditory stimulation of the stabled equine: The effect of different music genres on behaviour. Hartpury College, Centre for performance in equestrian sports (2012).

Rock 'n' roll music is a music style that originates in the rebellion of the youth with powerful vibes that stimulate the excitation of the brain. It is well-known that during rock concerts, in the 1970s, teenagers used to place a raw egg on the stage, which would be hard-cooked by the end of the concert by the strong vibrations produced by the music.

Also, an Australian physician and psychiatrist, John Diamond, showed that rock music caused a switch in the brain that caused a dissymmetry between the two cerebral hemispheres, causing muscles to become weak when subjected to the "stopped anapestic beat" of music from rock singers and bands, such as Led Zeppelin, Alice Cooper, Queen, The Doors, Janis Joplin, or The Band. Rock music would also lessen the abilities to work and learn. And according to a research done in 1968, plants would even wither and die when submitted to rock music.

On the contrary, classical music seems to be the most beneficial for our health, most probably also along with religious and relaxation music. Classical music lowers the heart rate, blood pressure, and fosters sexual arousal.[45] For a long time, there has been much marketing done about what has been called the Mozart effect, which would allow an increase in the IQ and studying abilities.

People rushed to buy CDs for babies, teenagers, and old people thinking it would develop their mental capacities. But

---

45 St Lawrence JS and Joyner DJ. The effects of sexually violent rock music on males' acceptance of violence against women. *Psychology of women quarterly* 15 (1991): 49–63.

it has been since demystified and proven that Mozart music could make the IQ raise by three points for only 15 minutes after hearing the music, so no need to play the "Kleine Nacht Music" in a loop all day and night long, it does not work!

In the end, it would seem that a beat of 60 times per minutes would foster concentration and enhance learning abilities whatever the kind of music.

A Bulgarian psychologist, Dr Georgi Lozanov, used this technique to create a revolutionary learning method for foreign languages, which he calls suggestology. School students would learn in one day 1,000 words of vocabulary and would have a recall rate of 92 percent after that day. Four years later, without further learning or practise, they could perfectly remember these 1,000 words! And that was done with a special 60 beats/minute music pieces.

Music is a direct communication to our mind and spirit and being aware of the choices we make is already a great step towards finding background music that is beneficial for us. Also, when you are going out to a cafe or restaurant, you will immediately analyse your feelings and know that a sudden stress or urge to consume might be well be triggered by the music that is played in the premises.

You will notice that in big shopping malls or supermarkets, in addition to the loud, fast, beating music, all the lights, cables, and electrical networks under your feet, and above your head make you tired, suck your energy, make your mind blind and confused and push you to buy all the products you need (or not at all) as quickly as possible and leave the place. You might not feel anything today when you are at these places, but once you start a digital, technological, and physical detox, you might well feel it and cut your shopping expenses drastically!

Prayer and gratitude:
The ultimate food for my spirit

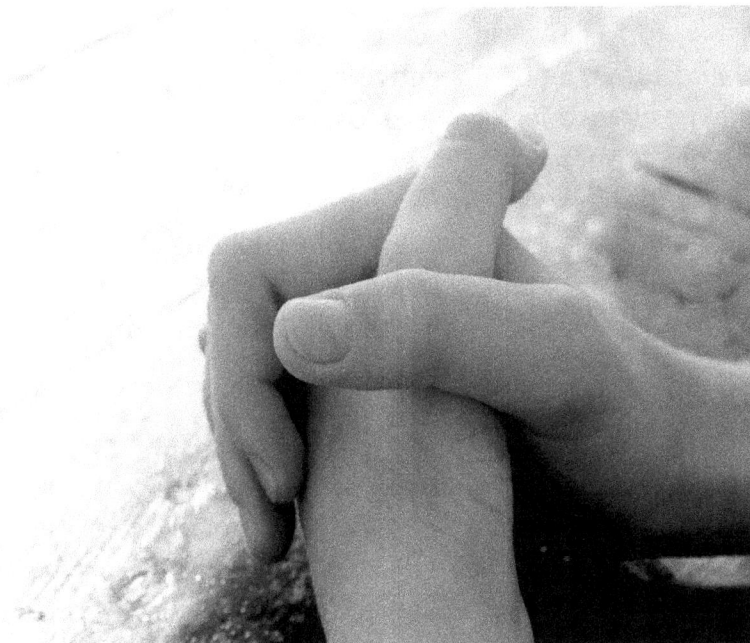

Remember Emoto's water crystal for love and gratitude? How regular and harmonious its branches are? Love and gratitude to ourselves will bring this harmony in our body as we are mainly made of water, but we might even think to our planet made of water for 70 percent, which will also benefit from our positive thoughts and the love and gratitude we express towards our universe.

We all know many examples of people who have everything for themselves but are not happy . . . you might even be one of these persons. Living near Monaco during the summer, I met many people who had a fantastic villa with a pool overlooking the rock bay, beautiful kids in the best and most expensive schools of the region, a nice car, a good job, lots of money to enjoy all kinds of activities and pleasures life can offer, but they were deeply unhappy. They were always lacking the next thing to be happy. They were angry and criticising almost everything around them.

I was for a long time angry at everything around me and would rather notice negative events of my days rather than the positive ones. On the contrary, you sometimes meet simple farmers or workers, often in remote and poverty-stricken areas, who are so happy and grateful for their life. Happiness is a decision, not a status, and practising gratitude is a great tool to achieve it. For everything can become a reason to be grateful and help this way to our energetic system to be harmonised also.

The Hartman institute studied practitioners of reiki, which is a meditative and healing Japanese practise, and observed that not only were these people happier on average than others, but also that their energetic body was perfectly aligned. A good moment to practise gratitude is in the morning when you wake up. Thank the universe for the day to come and say out loud to yourself "this is the day the universe has given me. I will be glad and rejoice in it".

Starting the day by declaring that your day will be full of joy and that you will enjoy it no matter what, is a powerful energetic tool. Keeping silent for a few seconds or a minute before eating, thanking nature for the food you have in front of you will be a great way to practise gratitude and increase the energy of the food as will be mentioned in the next chapter.

Journal of gratitude

To give a frame to your gratitude practise, you might want to write in a notebook especially designed for this purpose, five reasons to be grateful every day. If you want to practise it with your family, it is also a fantastic experience and you are so lucky to be able to do so. Before dinner, you might want to quote, each one of you, three reasons or things for which you are grateful. If you want to do it alone, you can write it down in this special notebook that you will be able to read months or years after it was written, which is always as interesting as it shows the ways you walked up to now.

It does not matter if you repeat yourself or often quote the same element. Your brain and your subconscious record the information, and the most important part of this exercise is to practise gratitude—to say the attitude of thanks, acknowledgment, and amazement towards life and the universe.

After my graduation, I had had a rough time finding a job and had a rather difficult break-up with a relationship at the time, which really brought me to a state of severe depression. Forcing myself to write every day five things that I was grateful for and which provided me a moment of happiness, made me realise how much pleasure I could take in small pleasures of life . . . which was not easy at the time.

I was often quoting things that might seem ridiculous, such as "ate a tasty tomato", "a nice person who smiled and opened the door for me", "my family", "my small studio flat", "the coffee I had in a nice cafe", quoting all these small things made such a difference in my life that I can only encourage you, especially if you are facing frustration, discouragement, depression, anger, or fatigue . . . to practise it. Buy a little notebook designed to be your "gratitude journal" and use one page per day.

Prayer, a successful style of life

Praying has become for many people in our societies an outdated and useless concept, if not something imposed by religious authorities or government to maintain social cohesion.

The prayer as a style of life that I want to mention is an essential food for our spirit and it is a personal prayer that comes from the heart. It is not dictated by an obligation or a show-off in front of others. The first and best prayer one can make is to practise joy and gratitude.

Prayer is before all a sign of gratitude to God or to the universe, whatever your religion or your belief is. If you do not believe in God, you can thank nature for everything it gives: get used to practise it in many situations, a nice flower you see, a beautiful cloud, a perfectly constructed building, your bus on time, a reduction you were given in a shop.

During times of need or illness, prayer is powerful not only to support us or the person we pray for on a psychological level, but also because it is effective and creates miracles. And when we pray, we enter the theta level of vibrations, which are the low vibrations produced by our body, bringing deep relaxation to our whole system.

Meditation is also an excellent tool to relax our mind and improve our health. Meditation, especially when spiritual, has some proven effects on the body, similar to those of prayer as it lowers the blood pressure, lowers the heart rate, increases the response of the immune system, and synchronises the cardiorespiratory system.[46] People who pray often tend to get less sick than others and recover better. A study conducted in the United States showed that people who never attended church had an average of three times longer stay in hospitals[47] whereas in Israel, heart patients were 14 times more likely to die following a heart surgery if not religious.[48]

You might think it is only a matter of being optimistic or happy and has nothing to do with spiritual or supernatural effects . . . it might be. But studies tend to prove that prayer is effective: Crawford took 45 clinical cases and 45 laboratory cases to evaluate the effects of prayer: 70.5 percent of the former and 62 percent of the latter reported a positive result on the samples (people) who received distant prayer and healing (reiki).[49]

---

[46] Various sources such as Cysarz D and Büssing A. Cardiorespiratory synchronization during Zen meditation. *European journal of applied physiology* (2005). Springer R and Schneider et al., Meditation might reduce death, heart attack and stroke in heart patients. *American heart association journal* (November 2012).

[47] Studies quoted by Koenig HG, McCullough ME, and Larson DB. *Handbook of religion and health.* (Oxford: Oxford University Press, 2001), 317–320.

[48] *Handbook of religion and health,* 22.

[49] Crawford CC, Sparber AG, and Jonas WB. A systematic review of the quality of research on hands-on and distance healing: Clinical and laboratory studies. *Alternative therapy health medicine* 9 (2003): A96–104.

Prayer also works for animals! The advantage with non-human species is that results are hardly impacted by psychological effects or placebo. A study done on bush babies showed that intercessory prayer on wound healing during four-weeks time decreased the wound size and hematological parameters greatly improved for the primates that received prayers.[50]

I recall here the story of my sister's dog, Jana, who had eaten a processionary moth and was rushed to the veterinary emergencies with a fatal diagnosis: the dog had half of her tongue burnt by the poisonous animal, which was still active and destroying more cells on her tongue, which would bring the tongue to die and fall, making it impossible for the poor dog to drink or eat . . . the vet gave the dog a pack of antibiotics to stand the pain during the weekend, and 48 hours to live . . . following which he wanted to euthanise the dog.

Four people intensively prayed and interceded to declare that the dog would not die and would get new cells on its tongue, which still had poison on it, and was dying slowly. We also did two energy therapy sessions on the dog to remove the perverse energies and refill it with new energies. After 48 hours, the dog was back on its feet and the vet who examined it, in the end, four days later, could not believe that not only the poison did not expand and reach other parts of the tongue but also the part that had already burnt

---

[50] Lesniak KT. The effect of intercessory prayer on wound healing in nonhuman primates. *Alternative therapy health medicine* 12 (2006): 42–48.

and died appeared healed! He could not explain how such a big wound was reduced to a 1 cm2 wound, enabling the dog to use its tongue again and be saved.

I could mention here the story of my friend, Frida Coleman, whose daughter was born with only one failed kidney and was seen as a desperate case by the doctors in Switzerland who gave the baby only a few weeks to live . . . Now her daughter is 15 years old, healthy, with not only one healthy kidney but two kidneys! The medical team refused to present the case for international conferences as it is beyond any rational explanation and the scientific community would question the authenticity of all the scans, X-rays, tests, etc., performed on this baby. I could mention thousands of unexplained miracles, some small, some big, some from my daily life, some about finances, jobs, visas, etc. . . . this might be called luck, baraka, a good star, but sometimes coincidences and random happenings are so strong that we might have to accept that our world is not only material but has also a bigger dimension.

It is noted that scientific studies did not report a difference in effectiveness according to the religion of the person praying or the person prayed for. I personally noticed that the name of Jesus is powerful to heal and change situations, but different cultures use different codes and formulas, you should find what suits you best. I believe that someone with a kind and well-disposed heart, willing to see things changing around her or him, with the faith that these things will happen, will see amazing results of intercessory prayer.

How to pray ?

People wish to have a relationship with God but do not know how to pray. At the beginning of my journey with God, I did not know how to pray, I was too afraid to pray out loud in a group of prayer and I was rather limited to the corpus of an official prayer you learn in your childhood. Then, my prayer was a shopping list for God's supermarket, please God I need this, and I want this, and make that for this person . . . until I grew and could meet people who taught me about powerful prayers.

An effective prayer always starts by giving thanks for what you have as mentioned before, as gratitude opens your heart to receive peace in your heart and receive God's word to you or your inner intuition for the projects and problems you might be facing. A study released in March 2015[51] shows a link between improved health and spiritual well-being was at least partially explained by the role gratitude plays in spirituality: "it is the gratitude aspect of spirituality that accounts for these effects, not only spirituality per se". So gratitude has a central place in prayers.

Once, you have given thanks for things around you and in you, you can intercede for others and yourself, often asking for the best to happen in a given situation. A famous verse in the Koran says "you do not know if it is good or bad for you" and therefore you should ask for doors of opportunity to open for you and the doors that need to be closed to be closed now and forever.

---

[51] Mills PJ et al. The role of gratitude in spiritual well-being in asymptomatic heart failure patients. *Spirituality in clinical practice* 2 (March 2015): 5–17.

Also instead of asking, I discovered that declaring victory and success was much stronger than polite requests, such as "If it could be possible, please arrange the universe so that this thing happen" . . . it does not work like that. You must declare that NOW your children are protected, that you have success in your work, in your relationships, in your marriage, that your finances are in credit always . . . practise this habit of authority and you will see the changes.

For those who wish to do so, you can mention Jesus' name, which is powerful, in a sentence, such as "I declare victory over cancer for my friend X or Y in the name of Jesus now". For people who believe in God or in a creator of the universe, you can say in the name of God or the creator. Also, you should be sure that what you have asked for will arrive. Does not the famous biblical verse say: " If you believe, you will receive whatever you ask for in prayer" (Matthew 21:22)?

Asking for forgiveness and guidance for your life is a good way to conclude your personal prayer. Once again, you should find the ritual that is the most adapted to your belief and feeling. For what comes out of our heart and what we believe with strong faith materialises into our lives. You will find at the end of the book a few examples of prayers you might use.

Conclusion

Health, happiness, and well-being are eroded concepts where all kinds of businesses, concepts, and innovations promise you to find them quickly with a few dozens, hundreds, or thousands of dollars of investment. The reality is much more complex and the results never achieved with an "easy" solution. It requires for each and every one of us to try, think, read, and find his/her own recipe. But it requires above all constant practise. The food we provide for our mind is so important because 55 percent of the energy our body needs comes from the food we put on our plates, but the remaining 45 percent is provided by the air we breathe, the sun and light we absorb, nature around us, and thoughts we put in ourselves.

Creating the right atmosphere around us and in us will be the key to our well-being and happiness. And our happiness will enable us to be a blessing to our environment, like a snowball that brings more and more snow sparkles around itself. Happiness is contagious, and that up to the third level of connection, that is to say the friends of our friends.[52] It has positive effects on siblings living in the same area, on our coresidents (spouse, children . . .), and neighbours. Also, this mind and spirit food change attracts around us more and more people like us, and fewer people with negative behaviours, this is the attraction law. We create the world we live in to a great extent . . . this leaves so many options open to us . . .

_____

[52] Fowler JH. Dynamic spread of happiness in a large social network. *BMJ* (2008): 337.

Chapter 3

Raise Your Energy Up

Do you sometimes feel exhausted by the middle of your day, with an impression that your vital energy has been sucked out by noise, people, and a busy place you went to? Some other days, you can feel so much energy even though you ate little, had a long drive to go to a remote place from home (usually in the countryside) and had long conversations with friends there. Why is it so? Each place has its own vibrations and energy and so do people, food, and things around us. This is why when you meet certain people, you feel your vital energy has been drowned out, while other people make you feel so optimistic and energetic after meeting them. There is a constant transfer of energies between human beings and their environments. It is therefore useful for you to learn how to protect yourself from energy suckers (could be people or places), which will be explained in the next chapter, but before that, it is important to know how to raise our own vital energy to enjoy vibrant health.

As we get stronger and are able to maintain a good energy level, we are able to come out of a state of illness much quicker, and when we are healthy, we have even more energy and we can focus more on spiritual matters rather than worrying all day long about our material concerns. It is important to understand that each illness has its own level of energy or vibration. Which means that if the person modifies his/her resonance with the illness by increasing his/her energy level (by an appropriate treatment, appropriate diet, appropriate lifestyle, appropriate thoughts, and spiritual or physical activities), it is possible to come out of this state of sickness and regain health.

Also, each place has its own vibrations. In general, cities in the mountains, remote villages, and holy places have more energy than big cities. However, even some holy places surprisingly have low vibration levels. It just means that too many visitors are coming to these places, mingling and changing the energy of the place, lowering its vibrations. This is why so many mosques or synagogues are closed to the public in order to maintain the original vibration's level high. It might not be explained as such in holy books, but this is one of the "energetic" reasons behind it.

Churches also had a direction of processions a long time ago, which had been studied. There was a door of an entrance and a way to walk up and down the alley and aisles, which was energetic although designed that way unconsciously. These procession ways have been totally transformed in modern times, to ease the access of believers or to suit the tourists. The energetic level has also changed and can be low compared to other places. Some bad mouths even claim that people from high-ranking secret societies or the religious hierarchy have turned these good energies upside down, or that most churches are built on temples that use to worship idols or negative forces, but this is far from our concern, which is to find ways to increase our energy level and be in good health.

Some countries or cities have higher vibrations than others. It all comes back to the environment, people, and thoughts that are produced in this place as we have seen in the previous chapter. It depends on the energy present in the place: does it encourage people to work, do businesses? Do people enjoy life there? Is the sea or the mountain close by? Are people rather optimistic or depressed in this place? Is the government putting pressure on its inhabitants or supporting freedom?

Energy level of the place (in Bovis Unit)*

(The Earth as accepted by scientists according to their school varies between 7,830 to 11,000).

Dubai 8,500
Mecca 7,000
Kaaba 9,500
(the black cube Muslims turn around which is the most holy place in Islam)

Cairo 4,800
Giza pyramid 14,000
Ibn Tulun Mosque (Cairo) 12,500

Jerusalem 10,000
Lamentation wall (Jerusalem) 16,000
Oman 12,800
Gaza strip 4,500
Gaza strip at war times 1,500

Petra (Jordan) 16,000
Beyrouth 7,200
Jeita grotto (Lebanon) 16,500
Maaloula (Syria) 22,000

Algiers 9,000
Los Angeles (USA) 11,800
Paris 5,000
Notre Dame cathedral (Paris) 10,000
Paris Grand Mosque 12,000

Shwedagon Pagoda (Burma) 18,000
(holiest temple of Burmese Buddhism in Yangon)
Mount Everest 14,500

* Results obtained by dowsing.

If you compare Paris with Los Angeles or Dubai, you can easily notice that the energies of these cities are different. As you can see in the image above, Paris has extremely low vibrations, almost the same as the Gaza strip, where people have a poor quality of life.

It is mainly due to the foundations of the city, which was called Lutetia and was a marsh at the origin, to the frustration of the Parisians (French people are the highest consumers of antidepressants in the world), stress and obstacles to work and establish a business, bureaucracy mind, and mediocre quality of life.

Whereas Dubai or Los Angeles are near the water, with a good quality of life, a good working climate, and a positive mindset of the inhabitants, which can make the difference. Many scientists would argue that these measures are not scientifically proven as the Bovis scale, named after its inventor, was mainly used by dowsers. It is partially true and this is unfortunately the only measure that is available to us at this stage of research in quantum physics and medicine, which are at their beginnings.

Hopefully, we will have other measures at our disposal in a few years time, as quantum medicine has only started a few decades ago. What these results enlighten are surely what I had felt from my own observation in various cities, sometimes wondering why I did not feel well in a church or a mosque despite it being a "holy" place, or why I felt energetic while being in a special cafe in the heart of a big city.

If the place we live in and work in matters so much in terms of energy, we also have the possibility when it is not exactly the right place for us, to go around and find places that feed us with energy, whether it be in nature, in a special restaurant, a monument, a religious worship place, or the house of our childhood. These happy places are the first way to enjoy a good level of energy or even raise it up . . . we have to find what fits our personality and character. But we also have to use simple ways to reconnect us to ourselves first and to the nature around us to elevate our vital energy.

Connect to nature

Walking barefoot in the grass or by the water is a fantastic way to get grounded, evacuate used energies, and capture useful earth energy, which feeds us with negative ions necessary to our body, which is submitted to high positive charges with the electricity and electromagnetic fields existing in our homes and environment. However, it is important to find a place far from agricultural fields, underground cables, and city parks as the quality of the ground is not anymore what it used to be 50 years ago.

French researcher Pierre Leruse has extensively studied the benefits of walking barefoot in nature, and he quickly noticed that the quality of the ground was essential to provide positive effects on humans. Walking barefoot in a place that has cables dug into the ground or a lot of pollution inside the ground is more harmful than beneficial—as we become conductors of electromagnetic fields or pollution ourselves. For him, the safest place to walk barefoot is by the beach on the wet sand next to the shore.

If you have the possibility, walking once per week by the water will enable you to release the used energies of your body and bring you the necessary telluric energies. Not to mention than breathing ioded air is good for your health. If you do not have this opportunity, you can take a hot feet bath or a full bath with gross salt in the water, as it is the salt of the sea that accelerates this process of used energy release. Walking under the rain used to be beneficial as it frees negative ions, but once again, the rain we get in our civilised world is filled with polluted, small particles that are harmful, so always walk with an umbrella above your head!

You might want to exercise twice per week by walking in a park or in a forest which is already good for your health as it gives oxygen to the muscles and frees dopamine, the accuracy and happiness hormone.

Eat organic food

Organic food is not only better for our health because it contains less pesticides, fertilizers, and additive ingredients than the traditional food found in our supermarkets, it also has higher energetic vibrations, which feed our body and mind with more vital energy.

Organic ingredients measured with the Bovis scale[53] show a higher score than traditional ingredients. Organic vegetables usually have a vibration of 1,500 BU higher than conventional ones, around 8,500 BU for organic vegetables against 7,000 for conventional vegetables.

Some processed foods have low vibrations, which sucks your vital energy instead of giving you some. In general, as we

---

53 Bovis—named after French radiesthesist André Bovis (1871–1947), the Bovis Scale provides a measurement of how positively or negatively a substance is charged.

mentioned before, fruits and vegetables have higher vibrations than meat, fish, and all animal products.

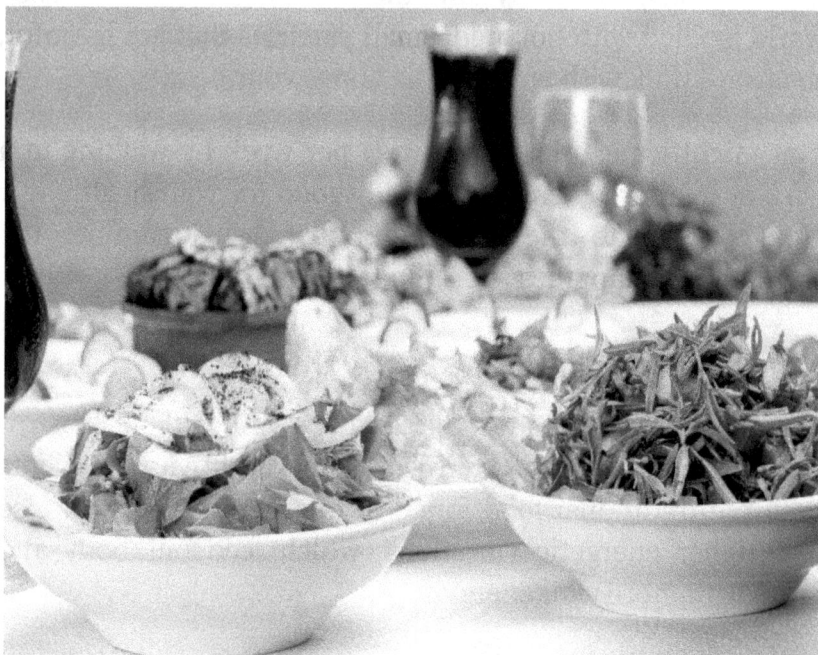

However, we can get even higher energy for our food when we inform it or magnetise it as the table in Chapter 1 shows. You can sometimes eat the finest and most expensive food, but if it is done with bad ingredients or bad energy, or with an angry cook, it will be empty, usually meaning you are hungry half an hour after eating. Exactly like a big beef burger and fries at the most famous fast food in the world . . . you feel so full after your meal, but you get hungry one hour later. Did it happen to you?

Talking about negativity, I used to know a lady who was so angry and depressed that all the food she used to prepare, although from the most expensive organic shops, was just disgusting and tasteless. On the contrary, I have some friends who have little money and cook simple things but you just enjoy being invited to enjoy such a feast of simple tastes, which means there is more to food than just the ingredients.

Everyone has their own experience and should find what suits him/her best in terms of food, but we have to bear in mind that there is more than just ingredients and calories in food . . . there are higher vibrations that we can call energy in the common language and they refer to the more subtle layers of vibrations present in the food, which are bringing us the necessary vital energy.

Show gratitude before eating

Showing gratitude before eating your meal, by observing a moment of silence or by giving out loud thanks to the universe or God for the food in front of you and asking for these nutrients to give the best information and energy to your body, will enable the food to have a higher vibratory level. Also, you can put your hands above your plate or the dish you are eating and ask the universe (or God) to withdraw all negative energies from it, all the animal suffering, all the bacteria, thanking the nature for its plants and products, and ask for its vibration to rise.

This will not only calm your mind and enable you to eat at peace and more slowly (which fosters good digestion) but also raise your energy level and the energy level of your food. In many cultures, it is customary to pray or give thanks before eating, which aims at blessing and informing the food present on the table.

Protestants pray before meals to give thanks to God and ask that the food would be full of energy for the body and spirit. Japanese say the word "itadakimasu" that means "I humbly receive" addressed to the cook and the nature. Muslims say "bismillah", in the name of God, each culture has its tradition. A friend of mine uses the Hawaiian wisdom tool Ho'oponopono[54] (that you will learn in next chapter) with her children saying sorry, forgive me, thank you, I love you for the earth and animals who produced the food . . . you can find your own ritual and adapt it as it suits you.

Energise the water you drink

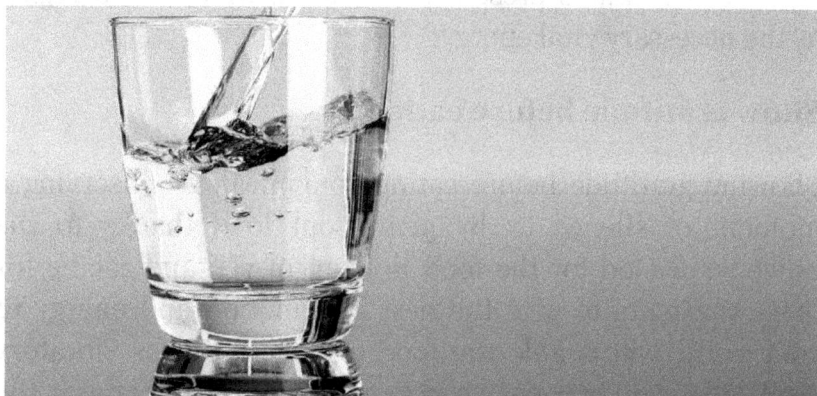

The water we drink loses its properties along its way to our glass. Tap water has lost all its properties by the long way it has been through in pipes, and the treatment it has been through to be drinkable. Bottled water also loses most of the nutrients and minerals that it has at the source, so you need to energise it.

---

[54] Vitale J. *Zero limits: The secret Hawaiian system for wealth, health, peace, and more.* (2008). Many other good texts have been published about Ho'oponopono, such as Duprée, Ulrich E. Ho'oponopono: The Hawaiian forgiveness ritual as the key to your life's fulfillment. In French Bodin, Luc. Ho'oponopono (Jouvence Publishing, 2011).

First, you can energise your water by shaking the bottle for 30 seconds, which frees negative ions, and you can add organic lemon juice inside to increase its energetic level.

You can remove the information contained in the water during its transportation by putting it in a glass bottle under the sun for two hours.

You can use the decagon symbol [55] available at the end of this book to inform the water you drink with the words or the remedy you want to provide for yourself. You can stick words inside the shape and leave a bottle of water (or oil) on it to which you will have carefully removed the label tag (which contains its own information).

You should leave the bottle on the decagon symbol for at least one hour in order for the information to get registered in the bottle, although you can just leave your bottles all the time on the shape. I usually put words such as peace, joy, or love, but you can write other characteristics, such as patience, focus, forgiveness, or a homeopathic remedy, such as "nux vomica", which is a current remedy for nausea or overstressed people.

Masaru Emoto and Jacques Benveniste, mentioned earlier, have worked on the information contained in water. Even miles after the information was given to the water, it still carries out the same information. The Korsakov homeopathic remedy works on the same basis. A tube that has been filled with one drop of the remedy and 99 drops of

---

[55] Annex 1.

water is washed 100, 200, 10,000, 100,000 times according to the strength needed for the remedy . . . we easily understand that there is no physical trace anymore of the vegetal or mineral used to produce the remedy after so many washings and dynamisations . . . but these highly diluted doses are effective to treat psychic and mental states.

What is transmitted in the remedy is information, not a physical substance. Water transports information, positive or negative . . . in cities it usually runs into closed circuits meaning that it keeps and adds the information turn after turn into the circuit. So you better desinform the water before consuming it!

Also, whenever you have the occasion, you can drink water from holy places as its vibrations are usually high but you have to check first the drinkability. Someone recently brought me a bottle from Lourdes, which is one of the most famous pilgrimage places in France, and its energy could be felt two meters from the bottle! A mineral water from the local supermarket prior to any energetic action usually has its energy level at 30 centimetres. Zamzam water in Mecca and Jordan River water have the same effect and so do all waters of holy places around the world, but our modern civilisation has brought pollution to many of them, making it unclean for consumption, so you better check if the water is safe drinking water, as you might otherwise experience some gastrointestinal disorders . . .

Breathe and recharge yourself

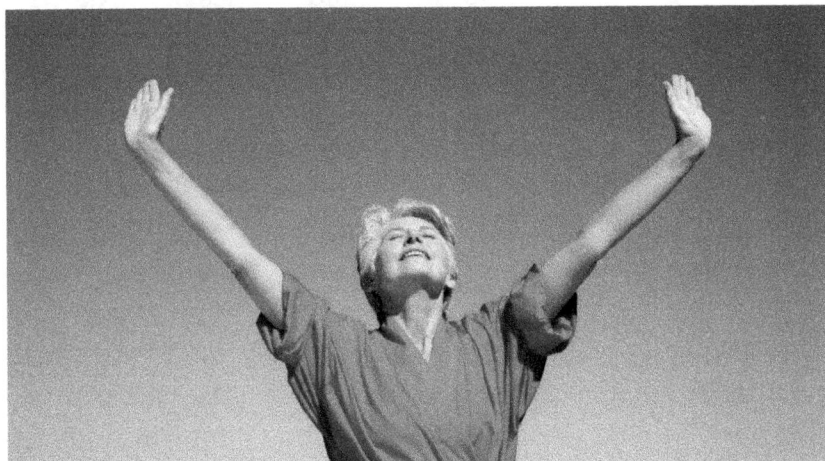

Breathing is what defines life. As long as we breathe we are alive, but we rarely pay attention to this amazing gift, which is a powerful tool to relax and recharge your energy. Every morning and every evening, taking a few relaxing breaths will enable you to start your day without stress and sleep well.

During one minute (which is approximately four breaths), you breathe alternatively from your left and right nostril while blocking the other side with your index finger. You should take as much air as possible when inhaling and you should hold your breath for three seconds and exhale slowly until no air is left in your lungs.

This alternative breathing enables your right- and left-brain hemispheres to be balanced and function equally. If you notice, you will feel more ease for one side or the other, depending on your predominant brain hemisphere. It is usually the right nostril that can breathe with more ease for women who are more intuitive and emotional. While it is usually more the left side for men who are more rational, relating to the left and right brain functions, but again it fluctuates according to your mood and worries of the day.

Once you have done this alternative breathing, you can carry on with five normal long breaths, each time holding your breath for three, five, and seven seconds according to your lung capacity, exhaling all the air contained in your lungs and blocking your breath again (for three, five, and seven seconds) before breathing and taking air again.

At that point, you should now distinctively get all the smells present in the air around you. If you have the chance to do this exercise near the seaside or in nature, you will smell the iode, the pine-tree essence, humidity, earth, but also if you are near a city, the car smokes or food smells, which you were totally unaware off a few minutes ago. You have now achieved the fast track to relax and recharge your vital energy.

However, if you can add three more steps you will really feel your energy level raise and get a deep sense of peace and unconditional love surrounding you.

We can mention here that some Christian people lift their hands during the worship songs of the religious services, capturing here the spiritual energies with their hands. Muslim people, when praying, put their hands perpendicular to their body palms up toward the sky, or they raise their hands above their breast before bowing down to the ground with the forehead connecting to the ground, which unconsciously enables them to capture cosmic /spiritual energies and be "grounded".

You can join your hands together in front of your breast and remain like this for a few seconds with a grateful mind. In

Japan, this sign is called gasho, which means "palms of the hands placed together" and is widely used by reiki practitioners before a healing session or during mediation but also by people of various religions. Asian people use it in their daily life to say hi, thank you, etc. Gasho is a fantastic tool to balance the energetic bodies, get grounded, and raise the energy of your body.

Doing these exercises usually raises your energy level a few thousands Bovis units, 1,000 to 5,000 according to some people, bringing more focus, more consciousness, and more peace and unconditional love for ourselves and the world around us. In the hectic world we live in, taking time for ourselves every day in order to be relaxed and raise our energy level is not a loss of time, but rather helps us to save time as we become sharper, confident, and communicate a good mood mind around us.

Capturing energies

Seated upright in a comfortable chair with your feet planted in the ground or standing on your feet, palms on your knee or leaning against your body, you imagine that you have energy going down through your feet and what is called the root chakra, located between your legs on your genital organs. The best way to do it, is to visualise many roots (like a tree) going from your feet and from the root chakra down into the earth, helping you to be fully grounded, a bit like a metal statue which is so heavy that it is rooted in the ground.

If you are doing this exercise in a building above the third floor, it is better to go down and do it on a plain ground, preferably not above a metro or underground car park but directly on sand, soil or the asphalt.

The second step aims at capturing cosmic energies. You can lay your hands palms up on your knees or perpendicular to your body if you are standing. You then ask to receive cosmic or sky energies in your hands and through your coronal chakra located at the top of your head in the middle of the skull now. You should feel like a white light and something heavy coming into your hands and your head. You should immediately feel peace, calm and relief in your body. This white light goes down to your heart when breathing and gets distributed throughout your whole body, organs, members, blood vessels, muscles, when exhaling.

If you do not feel anything, it is most probably because your left brain, the rational control, tells you that it does not work and that you do not feel anything. You should shut it down and try again while focusing only on the exercise. You also have to ask, as without asking it does not work: "I now ask to receive cosmic (sky, spiritual, heaven, celestial, God, holy spirit fire as you see fit) energy through my head and in my hands".

Chapter 4

Get Rid of Negative Energies

Marc was a lovely, energetic and confident guy who came to see me for a new diet program. He had tried out different diets, tried to eat healthy food, do exercise, he was practising spiritual activities, he seemed to be rather an optimistic person but it seemed that nothing worked to help him lose weight. He felt he needed something new. As we talked together, it clearly appeared that his diet or lifestyle was not so much the cause of his overweight and health issues but rather that his close links to his family, his anger and grudge against them was the cause of his acidity (or acidosis) and overweight . He was overloaded with negative feelings, which were like heavy suitcases that he needed to get rid of. We worked on cutting the emotional ties and practised forgiveness. In six weeks, he lost eight kilos without changing his diet. These exercises are quite easy and can be adopted by everyone.

We need to pay attention to our food, thoughts, and lifestyle to enjoy health and well-being, but first getting rid of emotional burdens and negativity in ourselves is essential to grow up spiritually.

Break free of emotional ties

In many cultures, family is so important that you should sacrifice your well-being and life to take care of your family. This was the case for Marc, who had from his young age taken responsibility for his younger siblings while his parents were working. They also had immigrated to France and he was quickly responsible as a child to do all the administrative work for the family as he was the only one to master the new language.

One of my Syrian friends dedicates her life to her family who stayed in the country. Being the only one outside the country, she has to use every penny to pay for medical interventions, medicines, and sometimes food for her mother, her brothers and sisters, their spouses, putting her in such financial pressure that I still wonder how strong she can be to cope with her situation.

Many Syrian people and others who come from a developing country or a country at war have to face the same situation, often becoming "a mule" where all responsibilities and pressure is loaded on them. Although it is morally hard and difficult when one lived all his/her life for his/ her family (their parents, siblings, spouse, children) to break emotional ties, it is necessary to do so in order to be less affected and become neutral to the situation. We do not mean here to break the contact, or love, or financial support, but only to break the emotional tie inside us, which makes us suffer. Once the ties have been cut, you will feel so much relief and freedom that you will not regret it.

I recommend doing this as well with past relationships, as soul ties have been established and remain, although we broke up or divorced a long time ago, sometimes we are even married with children, and these soul ties are still present, even though we are not in contact with the person. So it is necessary to close all doors to the past.

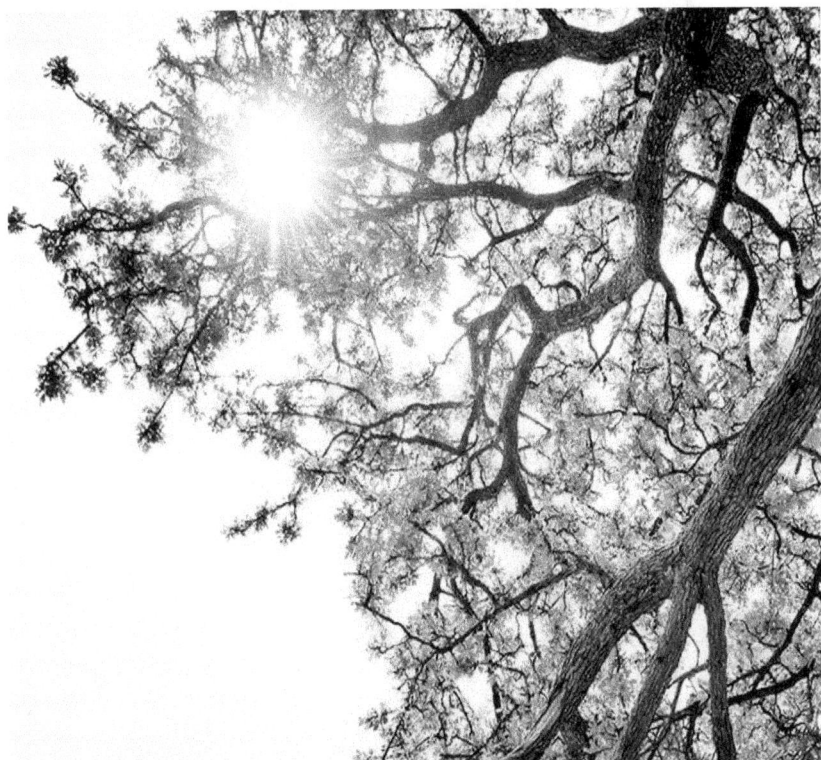

Moreover, it is necessary to cut ties with the family members who have passed away. It is not good for someone to cling to someone deceased and you are also hindering their way in the afterlife. My own mum was 62 when she finally accepted the death of her mother who died when she was 20. She let her go, freeing at the same time all the sadness and anger she had towards this event. She also did the same for her father, forgiving him what he had done, and the cruralgia (which is a deep pain in the front of the leg) she had felt for two decades without any medical solution, left her forever that same day. What we hold in ourselves in sometimes powerful and makes us suffer a lot.

The tree, the white rope, and the scissors

Find a tree you like next to your home; you might already know which tree you are thinking of, or you might go to a park or in nature to find one, in order to cut ties with the person you are attached to. If you cannot go out of your home, or it is hard for you to find a tree, you can just visualise yourself being under a tree. Close your eyes. Once there, you imagine that you see the person and all the situations you suffered from and all the things that are affecting you today. You then decide to free your forgiveness: "I forgive you". It might be very hard to say it, but once it is done you will feel so much lighter.

You visualise then, cutting the rope which attached you to this person with a big silver scissors. As you do it (you can use your hands to do the scissor gesture), you say:

> "I don't owe you anything.
> You don't owe me anything.
> You are big enough now.
> I let you go on your way of light;
> And I now go my way.
> I take what belongs to me, and
> I give you back what belongs to you (your story, problems etc).
> We are even.
> This is done now."

You then visualise the person going in the opposite direction from you, you can turn yourself back and start walking with the tree to your back, imagining the person is gone in the other way.

Cutting the ties under the tree is one of the most powerful tool to feel peace and freedom. But it has to be done with a forgiving heart. For some of us, we are not ready to do it immediately. We might have to do all the coming exercises before being able to cut the ties under the tree. Do not feel bad about it as it is normal. Do this as it makes you comfortable.

Write a (fictive) letter to the person you are angry at

There are many situations in life where we could not say what we think. Sometimes, we are not even in contact anymore with the person or he or she might be dead. Sometimes, it was even so traumatising that we could not raise our voice. And in some cases, the event has been for long, part of our unconscious given the violence of the shock experienced. It is often the case for rapes, sexual or physical violence, mental violence we experienced, etc. In that case, writing a letter where you say all you want to say to that person, especially what you are feeling inside you, is a powerful way to let your emotions come out. Once the letter is written, you can put it in an envelope and post it with the first name of the person (it will be collected and immediately destroyed by the postal service), you can put it in a river and visualise that all the pain, anger, and guilt has gone as it disappears along the flowing water, or burn it and watch the fire consume it. I like best the use of fire as it is a sign of destroying things but also of renewal and power.

Writing a letter to someone who has harmed you is difficult. I remember when I was a child that it was a real hardship, especially finding words and imagining what I could say to the person. But once you have done it, you feel proud and happy that you managed to do it. I can now mention it here without any hard feelings, which would have been impossible a few years ago.

Ho'oponopono, the Hawaiian reconciliation tool

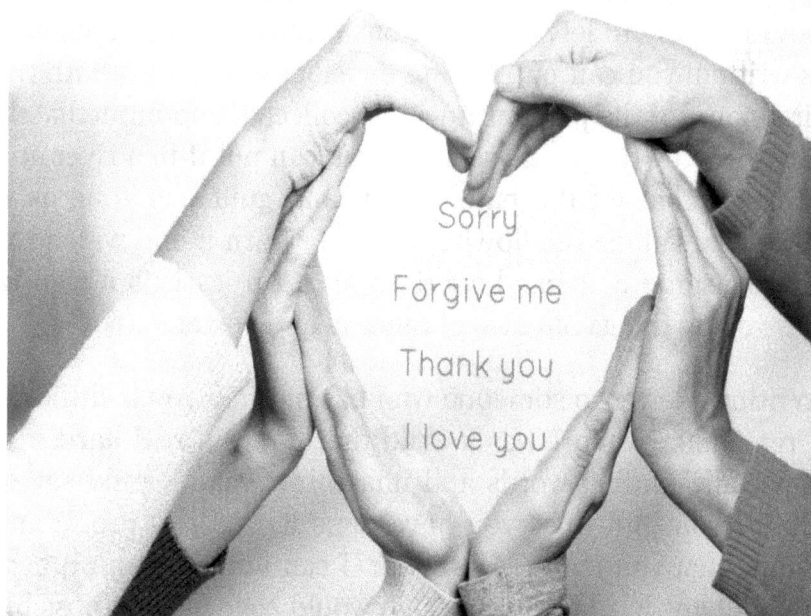

Sorry

Forgive me

Thank you

I love you

Ho'oponopono is a wonderful Hawaiian wisdom tool, which means to make right or correct what is wrong. It has been used for centuries in the community as a reconciliation tool when a fight opposing two people would be solved through this collective process of Ho'oponopono. A Hawaiian shaman, Morrnah, developed it as an individual tool and was even invited by the World Health Organization to present her findings.

But Ho'oponopono really became famous when Dr. Hew Len Ihaleakala publicised it and made it known throughout the world. He worked in a psychiatric centre in which there was a room dedicated to the mentally ill, criminals, and dangerous people. All the healthcare staff feared entering this room and was taking important security measures before entering it.

That is why Dr. Len could not get in to see his patients. He decided to study and work on their medical reports from his office. He worked on himself for the problems presented by his patients, and as he was working on himself, patients began to heal. They became less aggressive and treatments could be soon alleviated. Some patients were soon released and the unit closed within four years. When his colleagues asked Dr. Len how he could achieve such results, he replied: "It is quite simple, I heal the part of me that created them".

The Ho'oponopono process relies on the fact that we are 100 percent creator of our lives and that all things happening around us and to us are due to the erroneous thoughts that we have inside us. So if we want to change, modify, or improve things we do not like in our life, we must first understand and accept that we have created this situation. It does not mean that we have to feel guilty, but only responsible. I am not anymore a victim but an instigator because some of my thoughts are wrong and I need to delete it. I can act on it and others are not to blame.

Ho'oponopono:

Sorry

Forgive me

Thank you

I love you

Ho'oponopono is done through this simple process: we have to say these four words: "Sorry, forgive me, thank you, I love you". "Sorry" to be the creator of the event. I ask for "forgiveness". "Thank you" to life for showing me this erroneous memory I had in me and I was not aware of. "I love you". I love life, but mostly I send love to the wrong memory and I ask that it is erased . . . We might as well say, "I love myself" . . . Because Ho'oponopono uses energy of love to heal.

I would personally suggest writing up a list of people or situations that make you angry or events that have been shocking and hard to accept in your life. Do Ho'oponopono for a few days or weeks on each one of the persons or unpleasant situations mentioned on the list until the situation becomes neutral for you. Most probably, you will also notice some small changes in your life as a result of the process.

We do not do Ho'oponopono for a precise result, it is first intended to erase the wrong memories inside us, but it is also true that quickly, amazing results and changes in us and around us will be seen. It is also another way to clean negative memories, which I find more positive rather than writing a letter. But it can also be done as a second step once the anger and feelings have been expressed and released in the letter.

Once you accept that we are part of the universe and that our thoughts matter to make the world around us a better place, you will enjoy doing Ho'oponopono for many situations that do not concern you personally as the universe seems to be connected in one way or another in all its parts and you are a powerful actor in it.

Protect yourself

As much as you might pay attention to brush your teeth every morning, or put clothes on to go out, dressing up your psychological armour of light is important to protect your mental and emotional parts. To do that, you can imagine a big bubble of light (white, golden, transparent) from the top of your head to under your feet. You should feel that no one can penetrate this bubble of light and hurt you. You can say to yourself while doing so: "nothing forged against me can hurt me, for I am in the bubble of light".

If it is not enough and you are facing jealous people at work, for example, or nasty colleagues, imagine yourself being in a pyramid of mirrors. This pyramid goes from the top of your head down under your feet, in order that all negative thoughts, evil eye, and aggressivity will be sent back to the emitter. You might think that these tools are only in the imagination and they have no effect in real life but I can guarantee you that not only are they effective but also that what is done in the mind or spiritual realm affects the physical world.

Also, negative thoughts, anger, and criticism affect the person carrying these feelings. It might affect the person's mind but also his/her physical body, as negative thoughts can create illnesses. Therefore, we should try as much as possible to cleanse ourselves of negativity, free ourselves from guilt, anger, criticism, revenge, and disappointment, as by being angry at someone, we hurt ourselves more than the person we might have shouted at.

I used to fight with bus drivers, train station officers, tax collectors, and administration officers, but all the harm I was directing at them was directing back to me and was not solving the issue. Sending aggressivity always comes back to us. As I started working on myself and doing Ho'oponopono for the unfair situations in my life, I noticed that I was facing less unpleasant situations and that many situations got solved as if by miracle.

Cleansing the house and the room you are in

Whenever you are moving to a new home, whether for a short or longer period, you can use these techniques to clean the place from the energies that were there before. It can be positive or negative energies, but it is not your energies, so it is necessary to do a cleaning like you would clean the floor or remove the dust.

First, when moving to a new place, you can place cooking sea salt at the corners of each room and leave it there for a few days. You will then take it out with the vacuum cleaner, or give the floor a sweep and flush it in the toilet or in the garbage, but it is preferable to throw it into running water so it can be dissolved. You will pay attention to empty the bag of your vacuum cleaner and not leave the sea salt lay inside. Sea salt has been used since antiquity in different cultures to rebuke evil spirits and negative energies. In many countries, especially in the Maghreb, people put salt in front of their door and windows to ward off negative energies and purify the place.

You can also use incense, preferably what you burn on a charcoal, as it is of better quality, and leave it in the room you want to clean. You can buy it in a religious institution, whether Christian, Muslim, or Buddhist, as they usually have good quality incenses. All cultures and religions use it: you just need to go to a Buddhist temple or mass in a Catholic church to see that incense is used during the ceremony to spread out negative energies and elevate the souls to spiritual energies.

One of the most powerful cleansing techniques, used in drama techniques, is Michael Chekhov's method of acting, also used by energy therapists. It is to use an arm of light and sweep out the room with it. Russian drama techniques teach students to clean the stage where they are playing with imaginary arms of lights, and all together they take the old energies out of the stage. Each one of them washes the air with his/her arms and takes out the old energies, which they gather at the centre of the room until they carry them, like a bunch of dirty towels, out of the place.

Energy therapists open their arms and start from an extremity of the room and imagine they have white or golden arms of lights, which take out all the negative energies of the place. They then open the window or door and make a movement to throw these energies out of the place, asking the universe to transform it into energies of light and love.

These techniques might seem a bit ridiculous for concrete people who do not see the influence of energy in their world, but I can assure you that once you see how effective it is, you will use it wherever you are, especially in hotel rooms, which might have been used by all kinds of different people. Of course, if you are staying in a hotel, you might not want to place salt at each corner of the room, so you can just do a quick arm of light sweeping of the place.

Curses and entities

Until I became an energy therapist, I used to think that curses or evil eye were something of the African or Maghreban cultures, and did not really exist. I would always find it amusing that marabouts and all kind of magicians would give out their business cards in popular neighbourhoods of Paris and sell some special "remedies". However, the bad thoughts or evil eye that people sometimes send to others might affect their well-being.

Most of the time, health issues can be explained by the medicine and scientific knowledge. But in some cases, especially when people have irrational behaviours, fertility issues, periods which do not come, or lasting fatigue, it can happen that there is a spiritual explanation to it, when all other causes have been excluded. One should just be careful not to think too much to these spiritual issues, as we often attract what we are afraid of.

What you should know is that anyone engaging in activities to bring negativity to the life of others always get back what he/she sends to others as negative energies sent out, always come back. You should not try to take revenge, as the universe always will turn things around in your favour. Then, you should avoid being in contact with people engaging in these activities.

Also, you should try to live a life that does not attract negative energies to you. Tobacco, use of drugs, alcohol, prostitution, multiple sex partners, gambling, and excessive anger often attract negative spirits. It is like this negativity cloud that we mentioned earlier that people carry over your heads that attracts similar energies like a magnet. If your family was involved in spiritual activities that affect the well-being of others negatively, you should cut ties with the person involved, even if it is a deceased member, up to the third generation (your grandfather or grandmother).

You should first ask the universe (or God) for forgiveness for their activities and declare that you refuse the influence of evil forces in your life, and that you rebuke each action that has been done against people in the past and that you decide to walk in the light and path of positive thoughts. If you think you are experiencing troubles linked to bad thoughts that have been directed to you, you can use salt, incense, cleansing prayers, and refer to a specialist to help you, as Western medicine usually cannot deal with these rather irrational issues.

But once again, people often tend to think that irrational causes are responsible for their lack of well-being, when most of the time they are just keeping negativity alive around them by having negative thoughts, jealousy, anger, or lack of forgiveness themselves. We are creators of our life and watching our behaviour and thoughts is essential to be happy.

The ball of light is powerful

As we grow spiritually, we notice that not only do we need to eat well, have a healthy lifestyle, and raise our energy, but we also quickly realise that sometime dark stains on a white sheet do not disappear by rubbing it with strength, it only gets bigger and get more encrusted in the cloth. So, the stain must be carefully removed with a special stain remover, which will act locally and remove the stain.

Cleaning your bad memories as they come along is essential to enable you to be free. However, the strongest tool at our disposal once we have cleaned our mind, is forgiveness and love to our opponents. It might seem naive and weak not to retaliate, especially as we always heard that we should give an "eye for an eye, tooth for a tooth" but this principle does not free us from our own negative feelings, it is just a cosmetic solution that we offer to ourselves, which is encouraged socially by generations of people thinking this way. But as we need peace for ourselves, we can send love and light for ourselves but also for the person we are in conflict with.

To do so, we capture cosmic energies in our hands as we did before to raise our own energy, and we place our hands facing each other. We can now feel this aggregated energy, which is like a ball of light and we imagine sending it to the person we are in conflict with, afraid of, etc. . . . Chekhov's drama method advises actors to imagine that they are hugging and embracing the public, or a jury in a casting, to remove their fear and put the attention on the other who will feel happy and positive towards them.

Amazing results can be seen with this ball of light and love. I cannot name all situations that have been solved or the countless miracles that it has produced. I will just mention an anecdote as I was staying in a hotel near Disneyland two days before my own wedding, busy and stressed by all the preparation. The water in the hotel was ice cold, not to mention that the bed of the room was broken. The hotel was full and the management did not want to relocate guests or refund anything, despite the problem lasting for a long time.

As we were at the front desk to complain, there was a guy standing next to me who was getting angry and was asking for a refund . . . exactly like me. People behind us were shouting and I was in the mood to make a fight to get my money back. But I decided to withdraw and sit in the lobby doing my ball of light. You might not believe it but 10 minutes later, as the police entered to arrest and put in custody the guy who was standing next to me who got violent with the receptionists, the director of the hotel, came out of nowhere and asked me to come to his office . . . to give me a full refund for the night I had spent in his hotel . . . none of these other tourists or any other guest received a refund on that day, and I still don't know how the director came out to pick me in the lobby, but it just happened! I don't talk here about all the shopping and administrative issues that could be solved with it . . . it is countless!

The ball of light is powerful! Love casts out fear, anger, aggression, depression, guilt, and cleanses our hearts.

Chapter 5

Embrace Success and Happiness

Health and happiness is the normal state in which we should always be. It does not depend (solely) on external factors but it is deeply rooted inside us. In this perspective, illnesses or depression are only the signs or red alarms that our body is sending us to inform us that something is wrong and we are not on our path of life. It is funny to notice that in French, illness is said with the word "maladie", which can be written "mal a dit" (the pain has said) or "mal à Dieu" (harm to God). An illness is nothing more than harm that has been done to the principle of life and to our body.

On the contrary, when we put into action the principle of life, we start to heal and we can enjoy life again. Once again, in French, to heal is translated by "guérir", which can be also written as "gai" and "rire", which are "happy" and "laugh". Being happy and laughing are the best therapy to regain health, what many hospitals have understood by providing "laugher relaxation" classes and bringing in clowns in children's hospitals and cancer departments.

Our ultimate goal in the end is to find unity within ourselves and with the nature around us. Often, we are fooled into deceptive theories and practises, which promise us to find peace and harmony. But the plain truth is that happiness is to be in harmony with oneself and find this unity with our environment. And this unity can be found once we know our true identity, not the one people have given us or the one we try to build.

Identity and path of life

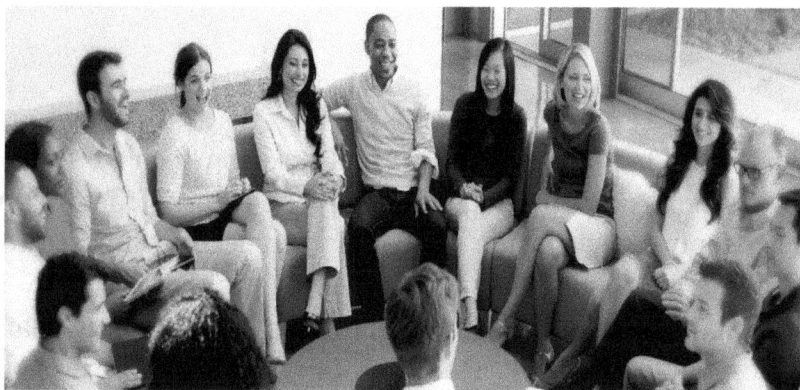

What is our identity? We immediately think to our name, date of birth, and nationality. These are the basic characteristics of our identity and it already conditions how we think, how we behave, and how people around us treat us. We all revindicate, in one way or another, our identity. The identity we build for ourselves is what we give value to and we want it to show from us. It can also be the result of early trauma, episodes of rejection, for instance, which will drag us into taking an identity that stands in opposition to what we have experienced. It is in this case a "rebellion identity". We all want to be acknowledged, to be "someone", belong to a category that we think will establish our value. This endless research for identity often lures us into deception or frustration.

As we can never be good enough. There is always something more to do, something more to buy, something to change or transform, something to get . . . Most people love so much the identity they are trying to build or have worked so hard to build that they cannot find this unity, harmony, or true identity that defines us. Also, most people work on one identity, the one they have been assigned by others for so long or the one they think they are. The risk here is that once this identity collapses, the person feels empty and can become depressed.

I remember the case of Claudia, a brilliant British journalist who grew up in Uganda. She was often saying that it cost her so much effort to be accepted as an English-speaking journalist of African origin. One day, she was contacted by an African channel that asked her to file reports in Swahili, her native language, which she did not speak well anymore as she had dropped it at an early age to integrate into British society. It was amazing to see how hard it was for her to be acknowledged as a good journalist but also as a black girl who lives like any other European lady, with the same passions, culinary tastes, clothes and style, parties, etc. Claudia was writing a blog at the time and was asking, "Where can I fit? As I tried so hard to be British and now I need to learn my own native language, work on my accent to fit again in the society which I come from and where I do not belong anymore."

This feeling of being neither this nor that and being between was also the case of my friend, Alicia, who is half Algerian, half Russian. On most occasions, she would take her identity as a Russian woman from orthodox faith, but she would sometimes be so happy to show her Arab origins by speaking Arabic with bus or taxi drivers, which would make her Russian friends feel awkward. This loss of identity and feeling of "in between", neither a native in their country of adoption, a foreigner in their country of origin, is a well-known syndrome of immigrants who do not know how to be themselves and adopt an identity that is not fully theirs.

The film of Algerian Mohamed Hamidi[56], Born Somewhere, summarises this quest of identity of immigrants and gives a wonderful analysis of the suffering this quest produces. My husband, Marc, fought for years between two identities, trying for so many years to be fully French and reverting excessively to the culture of his country of origin . . . . until he could find peace and harmony within himself. He now presents himself as he is, a person with a diamond identity, making the multiple cultures an asset rather than a lack of something.

Being as we really are without caring about others' opinion is such a blessing when we succeed in doing it. Other people put their identity in their house. Jean-Paul, an old friend of my mum, renovated a castle in the south of France and put all his free time for ten years into it, painting, decorating, renovating every inch of the place to make it perfect . . . until he started being ill three years ago. Many friends suggested selling the place as it was difficult to maintain, but he categorically refused, as this place is the only identity that he

---

[56] Hamidi M. Né quelque part (born somewhere) (Quad Productions and Kiss Films, 2013).

has. He is so proud to show every detail of the place to each visitor, and how he refurbished it so well, that without this place, he is nothing more than an uninteresting retired man who has no value, or so he thinks. People who have worked for years in a company and lose their job or retire face the same frustration or disappointment, as the only identity they had is collapsing.

I also have friends in Monaco who put their identity in the private school they send their kids to, the big SUV, the big LCD-screen TV, the pool, and the best restaurants they go to in the principality. They seem quite unhappy and miserable, but they are ready to fight for the image they have to present around them, especially that sometimes this standard of living is over their actual budget. So they work hard to pretend and present that this identity is the climax of happiness.

Another friend, Katy, has put her identity as an ill person. She regularly goes to the psychiatric hospital for a few weeks, goes out, always breaks her leg, or gets a bad flu that forces her to stay home and ask for some help. She desperately needs the love of others and has found that the only way people can care about her is by being ill and having health issues. Once she is healthy, the people who care for her, or are paid to care for her, such as the psychiatrist, doctors, and nurses, will not be there anymore. She fears that she will be no one anymore once she loses this identity. The identity she has built around sickness and hospitals could collapse if she changes her job, which she does not like, if she moves to a city or country where she has friends, and is more adapted to her lifestyle.

I could quote the example of Selma, a French student who converted to Islam and gets her identity through the devotion and kind of extremism she puts in her new faith. She likes to visit her family with full-covering clothes, telling other Muslims how to eat, how to pray, how to remove signs of their culture, which is not 100 percent Islamic compliant, and making fights at university to get recognised as a French citizen and as a Muslim.

It is true that her new identity has brought her a lot of new friends, through a community that has accepted her and sees her as special. She has also a lot of attention from French people who have a lot of interrogations about her faith or show signs of dislike for her lifestyle. She finds in her new religion the values and morality which she lacked in her family. In this case, it is a rebellion identity, a way to stand in opposition to what has hurt her and where she has been rejected.

This behaviour is unfortunately common among the young Muslim generation, which is not accepted as they are in Europe and decide to stand in opposition. They forge an identity and build a shield to be protected from aggression, avoiding looking deep down inside themselves, and healing the part of their heart that has been hurt. Other religions, political parties, clubs, and hobbies also try to gather a community of people who can find an identity there and become "someone".

All these persons, like you and me, try to have an identity that suits them. How hard it was for me when I left my job as a journalist to introduce myself! Who am I in the end? I quickly saw that the vision people had about me was different whether I was saying I was a journalist working for TV, or I am a naturopath, or I am unemployed. It took me time to realise that my identity did not lay in what I am doing, what I am wearing, or what I have.

I am a creature of the universe, a child of God who has a purpose on earth and in life. I try to be the best person I can, I forgive myself and I accept my weaknesses, I enjoy life, and I try to make the most of every situation, even when it is not enjoyable, as we always learn. Buddhists like to meditate in all aspects of their life, when they eat they eat, when they pray they pray, when they sleep they sleep . . . being present in each situation. It is a bit like the philosophy of Eckhart Tolle with the present moment[57] when we are here and now. Or the Ecclesiastes book of the Bible that says we should enjoy every moment of life as we are all going to die, just and unjust people also.

Finding our identity is our biggest challenge in life. The one that brings us the most happiness once we found it. And we often look for something external to fill this identity or this constant state of "lack" within ourselves as we look for it in places where it cannot be. We might be like Claudia, Mohamad in Monaco, Katy, or Selma, trying to achieve more, be more, buy more, or take pills to fill this emptiness or gap . . . but it will always be empty after a few hours or days.

As this empty gap that we have in our heart is designed to receive the divine part of us: whether we call it God, Holy Spirit, the divine part of us, the connection to the universe, total love, our higher self, unity with life . . . It is this feeling of being one, being in unity with ourselves and with what is around us that is important. Unity diffuses to all our blood vessels, cells, organs, and our mind and spirit. All the

---

57 Tolle E. *The power of now.* (1997).

elements and techniques mentioned earlier are only tools to achieve our real identity and unity.

Success, dreams achieved, and happiness will only be the logical consequence of this state of well-being. I encourage you to write on a piece of paper (honestly) the identity you have or that you use the most. You should then write five other identities that you have or five persons you want to be, as we are diamonds and should always carry different identities according to the situation we are in.

I wrote, for instance, "I am a person who helps people to heal. I am a good leader. I am an independent woman. I am a supportive wife. I am an excellent communicator". Find yours and review it as many times as you can, as by reconsidering it and declaring it, it will become yours. You are today the result of what you have been thinking about yourself for years. You can determine today whom you will be in the future by choosing to have the right thoughts about yourself.

Success and law of attraction

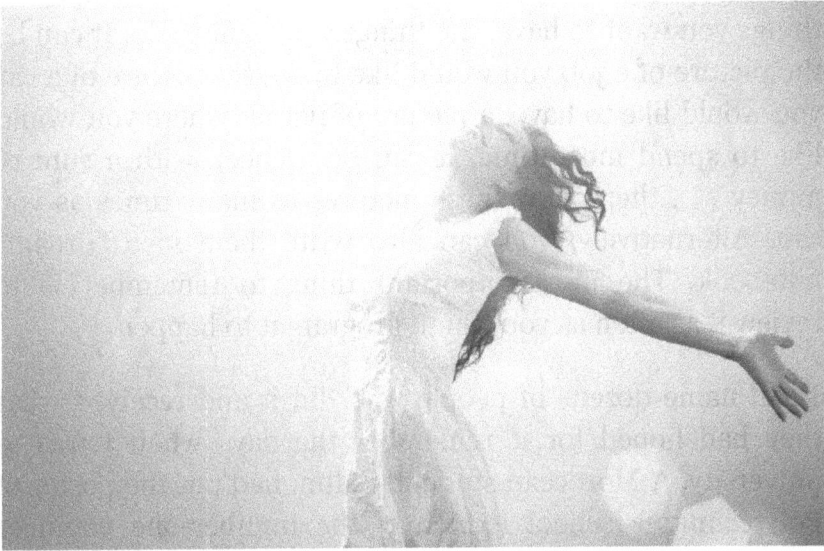

We are what we eat; we are what we think; we are what we give. Our daily routine determines whether we are and will be successful people or not. You certainly remember here what rich people do every day. John Maxwell, a leadership teacher, says "If I could come to your house and spend just one day with you, I would be able to tell whether or not you will be successful". And he adds to make people comfortable, "You pick the day".

Our attitude determines who we are and who we will become. Being successful, rich, and happy is a decision. We can take our dreams to the reality when we write them and watch them every day. This is what multimillionaires mostly do. Then, we need to speak them into reality as if they were existing, as what is hidden from us does not necessarily mean that it does not exist, it will certainly be there in a few months or years. Images are powerful to help us build our dreams.

Find a special box, (it can be a shoe box or wooden box), that you will call the "dream box". Put inside photographs of things you want to have, the things you want to do. It can be the picture of a job you would like to do, the picture of a car you would like to have, a picture of nature where you would like to spend more time, it can be a check with a sum of money . . . then, view these pictures as many times as you can. Alternatively, you can also write them in a "dream" notebook. The most important thing to remember is to review it as often as you can to program it to happen.

I can name dozens of people who did it and received what they had hoped for. I remember the days when I was at university. A Moroccan student, Salim, had put the poster of Polytechnique school (which is the number-one engineer university in France) above his desk in the small room allocated by the university. I was always wondering when I was passing in the corridor why he had chosen this big picture of the facade of the school with an ugly statue in front of it as an oversized decoration for his room. I was even more surprised that he decided to redo one more year of study when he failed to be admitted to that school and was received in the second ranking one.

It was so much work, and exams are so uncertain that for many students, it does not make much sense to do one more year of this intense preparation. But he believed that he would enter the school and was all day watching the picture above his desk. He finally entered the school the following year and he is now working as a top high-end stock exchange trader in London. Dreams come true and images are powerful.

Terri Savelle, who is a famous American coach and leader, says that she received the $100,000 she needed for her association by being certain that she would receive it in one year, looking at the picture of a check and praying for it to happen. So start visualising and believe that what you want is coming to you. Also, it is important to focus on what you want and do not focus on what you do not want, as our brain is set only on affirmative sentences. Do not say "I want my husband to stop ignoring me", but instead say "I want my husband to take care of me and be affectionate". Do not say " I will never have a baby", or "I will never marry", as it will set your brain to achieve what you say.

If you feel and say that you are rich, healthy, that you are a wonderful person, the universe will respond and turn things in your favour. This is why, by the way, you should avoid to say to a kid "don't fall off the chair" but rather " stay where you are", as the brain will certainly understand fall omitting the negative verb before it. Affirmations and pictures will help you there. And once again, do not stay in a position where you look at what you are or what you have today. For what you are today is what you have believed you were yesterday. Be sure that what you believe about yourself today will be what you will be tomorrow.

Reign over your life

Reign over your life means to behave like a king or queen in your life. It means to feel that we have the authority and power to decide about our life and our health. You certainly know rich people who think like homeless people and poor people who behave like billionaires. You might think when you see someone who is not so well off that he is showing off and should come back to reality. I do not talk here about people who unwisely spend their money and live over their budget. No, I mean enjoying a lifestyle of a millionaire because our heart is set to be rich and happy not because we throw money out the window to buy superficial objects.

The truth is that if we decide to live as joyful and prosperous people, we will enjoy life and reign over it. I once knew a Brazilian pastor in Paris who was addressing a large crowd of 5,000 people every Sunday in the city suburbs. When you saw him preaching and behaving in his social life, you would certainly think that he was an ambassador or minister of his country. Always driving the latest Mercedes car, well-dressed, speaking with confidence to everyone . . . the truth was that he was living in a small room on the sixth floor without a lift in a Parisian suburb, driving the Mercedes as a chauffeur and earning less than €1,000 per month. When I asked him about his secret to look so rich and so happy, he told me "I am living the life God has called me to live, which is joy and prosperity, and I have the faith to see things that are yet unseen".

The only difference between someone miserable or prosperous is in our thinking and behaviour. We are a creature gifted with free will, we can choose to reign over our life or think that others determine who we are and what we will be. This is the ace card . . . we can play it or decide to keep it for later, waiting for the right occasion to happen. The truth is that it will never be the right occasion, so believe and do it now.

Believe that you are prosperous and that everything is well in the world, which is yours at the moment. Believe that you have value and that you are on earth for a purpose. Believe that your life is meaningful and that you have the power to turn it in a way that satisfies you . . . reign over your life.

Finding solutions and making tough choices

There are many times when we are standing at a crossroad of our life, in a position where we have to make tough choices or we are facing an issue we do not know how to solve. First, you can write down your question or choices. Before going to sleep, for as many days that it takes to get an answer, ask the universe to give you an answer.

When we talk about hard choices, we are facing a choice where no alternative is better. It can be a choice of career: being a lawyer or an artist. One job brings more security and ensures an income whereas the other is more creative, with a lot of fun people around but is more risky financially. None of the options is best if we take it globally. If we exclude money or security, which are not equal to overall happiness, the artist choice might be better, but if we exclude the creative part of the artist job, we might well see more interest in a lawyer job. So this is a tough choice.

It can also be a question whether to marry person A or B. A is tall, handsome, intellectually interesting, and funny but does not earn money and is unstable. B is a bit out of shape, more traditional, but has a good income, and is responsible. Which one is best? It depends on which filter you apply to your decision, but it seems that a priori no choice is easy to make. Writing the positive and negative sides of each choice will not help here as one negative parameter can outset all the positive ones, or one positive aspect can be so important to you that you will be unhappy if you do not take this option.

Asking for help or a solution during times of tough choices will make your life easier. How? You will need to open your eyes, ears, and be aware of synchronicities.[58] As always when we ask, we receive answers if we can read it properly. Practising all the tools mentioned throughout the book, especially asking for a solution before sleeping and by having a healthy diet and set of mind, will set your mind to receive information that will help you to make a decision or to get a confirmation. To some people, it can be a voice that talks to you, or a dream, but for most of us, let's be honest, we will see signs.

I recall some American friends who were visiting France to find a place to live. They were due to go to Nice but an improbable technical incident happened and their plane was rerouted to Marseille, which is quite unusual as the city is 200km away from Nice. When they arrived there, they were not intending to stay even for a night, as the city had such a bad reputation. However, they saw a poster written in English: "Why don't you stay for real"?

A series of events happened during their stay that gave them a confirmation that it was the place they were meant to stay in. They have been living there for seven years now, their business has expanded, although it is not a prosperous place, their kids have a premium education although the city is quite poor, they have a wonderful flat in the city centre . . . only they could read the signs and synchronicities of life.

---

[58] Synchronicities are coincidences, events which happen one after another and do not seem to have any relations but make sense for the person who is experiencing them. Carl Jung defines it as a causal connection of two or more psycho-physic phenomena.

Closely watch the doors that are opening or closing for you, as things happen for our best if we are aware and observing them. You can use the request to the universe reminder at the end of the book if you wish.

Finding the right partner

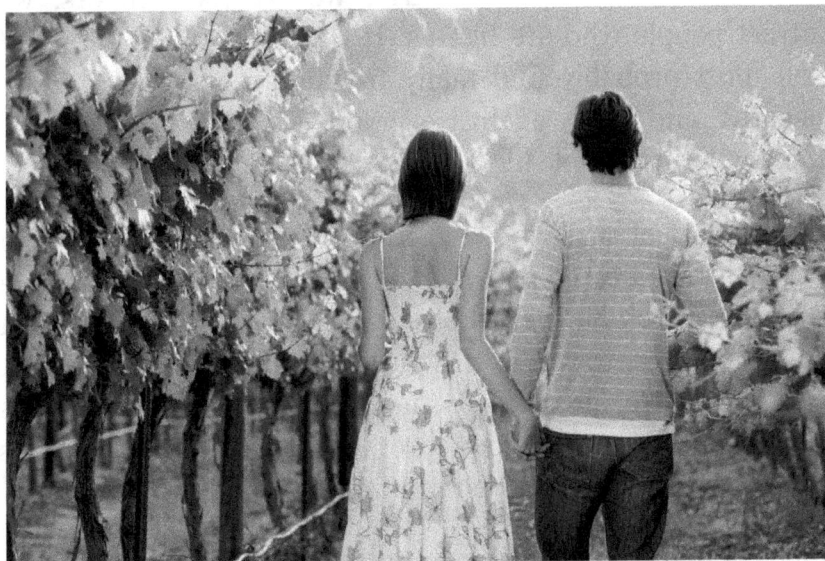

Finding the right person when you are single can be quite tough especially in a connected world where people talk less and are living in an individualistic way. In European countries, one third of people are living alone and the trend is developing in the Middle East and more traditional societies. Some are happy with it, others (maybe the majority) wish to find a partner to share their life with.

Meeting the right person is quite challenging, but it works more or less like finding a solution to an issue. You should ask for it. How? Once again by asking God or the universe to bring you the best person to share your life with. But before asking for someone to enter your life, you should be sure that you have already found your balance and happiness on your own, as there is no way that if you are unhappy with yourself, someone else will cover your unhappiness and make you happy. It will last for a while, but soon, the same issues you are facing will arise again.

Being found and knowing our true identity are key to meeting the right person. Also, we are like mirrors, we attract people who are like us. If I am a negative person, I will most probably find many friends around me who are negative and angry against everyone. If I bring joy around me, I will find people like that.

When we feel that we are ready to meet someone, we can write on a piece of paper all that we are looking for in a person. Write whatever comes to your mind, even things that you are too shy to say, as this piece of paper is only for you. It can be: tall, makes jokes, earns $10,000 per month, knows how to play the piano, good lover, eats organic food—write as many characteristics as you can think of.

Once you finish, you will post in front of each quality, D for desirable, E for essential. Then, look at the essential categories, and narrow the list to five qualities. The person you are looking for is that one and she might well be quite different from what you had imagined or what you would say you are looking for. Writing these five qualities and reviewing them quite often, like your dreams, will be of a great help.

It might be a coincidence, but a few years ago I had done this exercise and had written the five qualities I was looking for in a man. The true essential characteristics were quite different from what I would say to my girlfriends over a cup of coffee. I would tell them I would like a guy who is tall, thin, earns a lot of money, and graduated from one of the top three universities, whereas what I was looking for deep down was a generous, well-balanced man who loves himself and me.

Two months after doing this, I met my husband who has exactly the five qualities I wrote down, but he is different from the person I would have looked at a few months earlier. This technique has worked for thousands of people around the world, so just try it! Be patient, have faith, enjoy the small pleasures of life, and welcome what comes into your life with a positive heart.

Also, remember that we often meet the person who is the most suitable for us at the present time, meaning that our partner fills in the parts of us that are incomplete or gives answers to the issues we are facing. Which is why many people do not feel in harmony with their partner years later as they change a lot and, often, in a different way from the person they were living with.

If you are with someone you are unhappy with, you can work on it by using Ho'oponopono and sending light and love to your partner. You might not believe it will change something, but I guarantee you that things will change in a way you are not expecting. Whenever you get angry, frustrated, or sad, do Ho'oponopono and send him/her love and light. You have nothing to lose, it will make you feel better as you will not keep inside negative feelings and it will influence what is around you.

If you are unsure whether to get separated or stay with that person, once again, you can ask for synchronicities and signs to give you some answers. Meanwhile, writing your dreams, breathing, and practising good food for your body, mind, and spirit will help you get through this insecure or tough times.

My life is changing

If your life started changing since you started reading this book, it is normal and it is even a blessing. If you feel that it is hard for you to spend time with your mother or members of the family who tell you negative stories about themselves or give you bad comments about yourself, it is normal. If people who were close friends now feel that you are not the same anymore, or you do not have the same pleasure spending time with them, do not worry. You are starting to wake up and see things in a different way.

For the relationships you have had were corresponding to the state of mind you had until a few weeks ago and they do not fit anymore with you. And it will be more and more the case as time passes by and you walk on your journey towards more success, more peace, and more happiness. But do not worry, as the universe has placed people along the way who will be close to you, who you will learn from and grow . . . this is the resonance law.

If you have a passion that has stayed hidden for years, this is the right time to start practising it again, with a measured and adapted rhythm to your way of life, but do use your talents and feelings! Do something that makes you happy. If this is not possible at the moment and you do not find time to practise a hobby or passion, use what I call the "ice cream" moment. Five minutes per day, you should set on your happiness moment, which is something you really feel like doing for yourself, whether it is to eat ice cream, watch a funny video on YouTube, breathe clean air in a park, stand under a hot shower, buy a lipstick, eat fresh fruits, or try a new day cream . . .

Changes happen gradually. What is important here is to tune ourselves to the vibration of love, clarity, and happiness. You certainly remember the different energetic measures of foods, places, or the importance of thoughts. Being in the right place, practising activities and thoughts that enable us to have a vibration in accordance with the nature of the universe will immediately bring people and things that will be in resonance with us, as we are 100 percent the creator of our reality.

Once we get the first keys, doors start opening for us and a whole world starts revealing itself to us . . . with this specificity: it has no limit! So enjoy yourself, find your way, and expect the best to happen. Our only remaining challenge is to practise happiness and prosperity convincingly and violently. For our doubts and uncertainties hinder happiness. We sometimes like to complain, be frustrated, be angry, and repeat the story that has annoyed us for hours, but the truth is that we have to crash all this negativity. By spending time worried about money, health, or life, we create a blockade to the positive events that are on their way.

So, rise, shine, for the right day has come . . . now.

Annex 1

Water Information

Place a bottle of water (once you remove its tag) in the centre of the decagon, and put the words you want to inform your water with inside. Leave the bottle of water for a few hours to inform it with the vibration of the chosen words. It can be a feeling (joy, peace . . .) a remedy (aspirin, calcium, nux vomica . . .), an intention (protection, light, detox, digestion . . .) etc. . . .

A glass bottle is preferred, if possible, and you can first leave it two hours under the sun to remove all the prior information it had before coming to your home. Then leave it on the information plate below. Alternatively, you can place your bottle inside a circle you have drawn on a white piece of paper and leave it there for a few hours before setting it in the decagon.

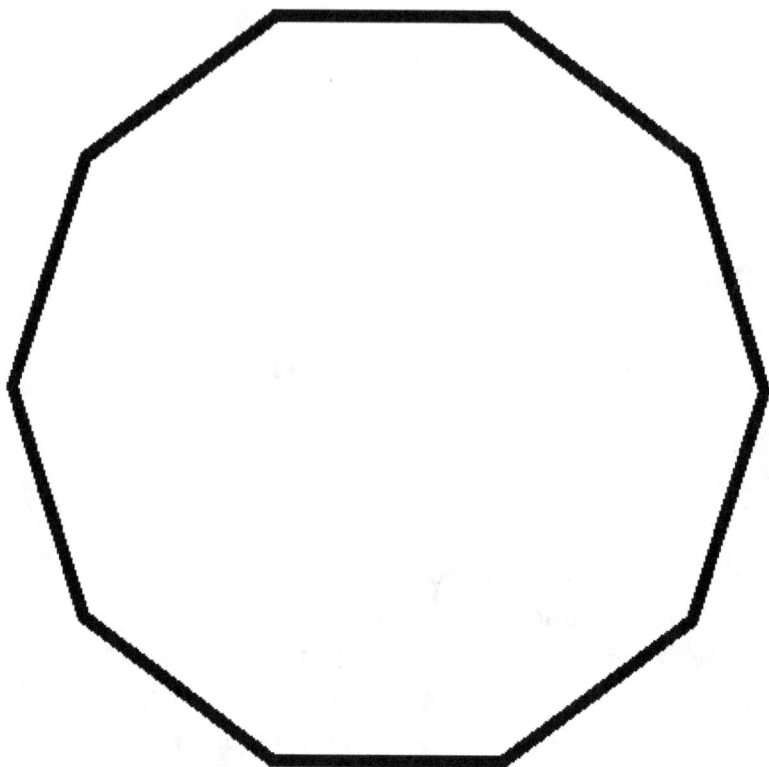

LOVE

JOY

LIGHT

Annex 2
Mono-Meal Ideas

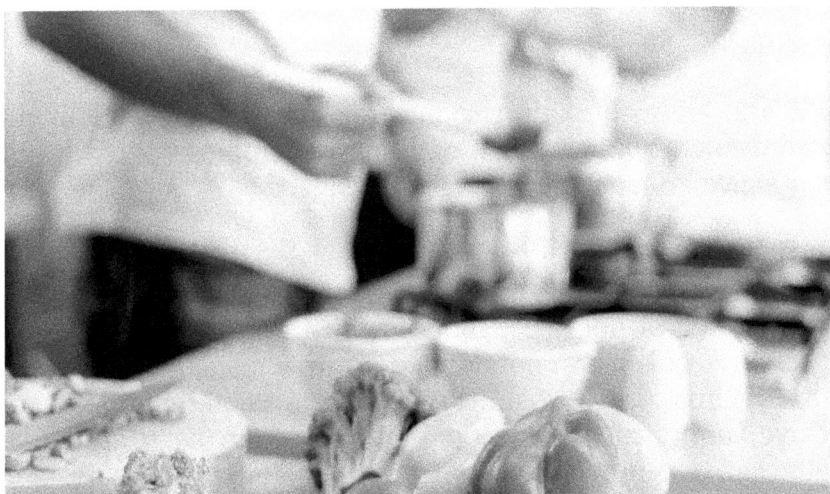

It is important to drink 1.5 to 2.5 litres of water according to your constitution, or herbal infusion (without sugar or with half a spoon of honey per cup) in addition to your chosen food. This mono diet of 24 hours contains between 650 calories and 900 calories for the day, helping you keep health and your weight, especially after a big meal, or if you had to eat outside your home during the week. Products should be organic, if possible, especially for that special day. You preferably do this once or twice a week.

Fruits

Choose one fruit and eat 1.5 kilograms during the day. You can do three to four meals during the day. Apples, pears, watermelon, cherries, strawberries, bananas, and grapes are good mono-meal fruits, but it can be any fruit available at that season and in your area. Grapes and bananas or other sweet fruits bring more calories. You can also do this mono meal with fruit juice. One litre of fresh squeezed juice or mixed juices during the day.

Rice

Eat 150 grams of plain rice in three meals: breakfast, lunch, and dinner. You can eat it with mashed apples, a little bit of soy sauce, tomato sauce, or a green salad.

Potatoes

Eat 3 kilos of potatoes, cooked with the skin on in a slow-pressure cooker or a pot. Served in three meals. You can add one yoghurt or soy yoghurt with herbs or condiments (basil, chive, mint, rose petals, or garlic, but no salt). You can alternatively add cumin and bake the potatoes in the oven or mash them. You can serve your potatoes with a tomato sauce, garlic and herbs, or with a green salad.

Zucchini

Eat 3 kilos of zucchini, prepared either as a soup (with an Aromat vegetable cube), as a salad (with one spoon of olive oil and half a spoon of nut oil, linen or sesame oil, added to a spoon of lemon or soy sauce), or baked in the oven with a bit of tomato sauce and garlic or onion. I suggest starting your day with the soup or the salad and baking your zucchini at lunch or dinner.

Annex 3
Useful Prayers

(You can say one of these prayers after your breathing exercises, before sleeping, or whenever you will feel the need to. For believers, you can replace the word universe with God, of course. I used the word universe to fit everyone's belief, but you should adapt it for yourself.)

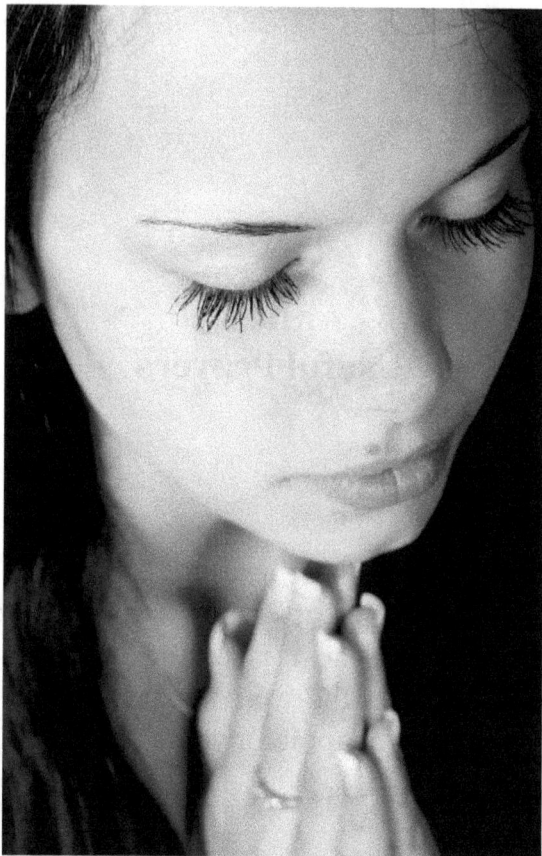

Prayer to the universe

I thank you for the nature around me. I thank you for life. I thank you for my health. I thank you for the healing of my heart. Thank you for the place I live in (even though I do not like it so much). Thank you for my family (even if they are imperfect). Thank you that each day I have food on my table.

I now free my forgiveness to people who have hurt me or annoyed me (today). I forgive myself if I made any mistake or if I am not perfect. I accept myself as I am, and I now erase all negative thoughts, ideas, and behaviours, which are in my mind. There is no negative feeling in me right now.

I ask the universe to give me signs and put the right persons on my way. That the doors that need to be closed, be closed now; that the doors that should open for me, open now. I want to . . . (have a job which I like, marry, heal, move to a sunny place, have a harmonious relationship with my family . . .). I know that my requests are heard and that I shall receive what I have asked for.

I decide to walk today in the path of light and love, as I know that the universe wants the best for me and that all my needs are met.

Prayer for healing

Dear Universe (or God),

I thank you for life. I thank you for health, which is here now (or that will be there soon). I thank you because you made my body and mind perfect.

There is no imperfection, no illness in the way you have created me, and I now proclaim that I am now completely healed, whatever the illness, the broken bones, the dysfunctional organs, the pain in muscles, nerves, internal organs, depression, and psychological diseases, I know that I am healthy and that all parts that have suffered are healed now.

All the parts of me that benefited from this pain or illness are healed now. My . . . (quote the part of your body that hurts, or your problem) is healing now, the pain is fading away.

I feel much better already, and I know by your mighty power that I am now completely healed and that I should feel it soon.

Prayer to diffuse negative energies of a place

(You should do the energetic cleansing with your arms of light first, and then say in each room the prayer, if needed.)

I now take authority over all negative energies, negative thoughts, evil spirits, and entities that are here. I order them to flee and go out of my home now. There is no place for negative energies here. I ask the universe (God) to protect this place, and bless all people living here or visitors who will come in this home.

Annex 4
Make a Request to the Universe

1. Write down what you want to have or achieve. It must be short, precise and clear.

"I want / I ask . . ."

"A doctor job at the Royal hospital."

"A flat with a balcony in Marina bay."

"A loving husband / wife."

"$1,000 savings this year."

"To be a confident person."

You need to write it down, as during our days many thoughts come to our mind and we cannot expect the universe to know what exactly we want. If you make a vague request you will get a vague result: "a job that I like" can be many things . . . try to make it more precise.

2. Review this request as many times as you can per day and ask God or the universe before you sleep to show you signs

and coincidences about how to achieve this dream or request.

3. Write a sticky note with the most important word on it and attach it to your computer, on the door, and on the fridge.

4. Be sure and do not doubt that the universe will answer your request.

5. Visualise yourself at the present moment in the situation. In one word, connect to your dream or request. Close your eyes, take a few deep breaths, and see the situation with your internal eyes—you at this job, you with this wonderful person walking in a park, you in this gorgeous house . . .

6. Also let the universe or God make the "how" of your request, you just focus on "what" you want. Do not ask, for instance, to meet your future partner through a dating website as it limits the answers. You might meet your future partner through friends or at an event. Or "I want to receive my aunt's inheritance to buy my house". Maybe the universe has other ideas on how to finance it, so leave the how open.

7. Be patient enough to see the result of your request.

8. Also, make sure that the request is what you really want and that you authorise yourself to receive it. Sometimes we want this dream job but deep down we think we are incapable of doing it, or we think we are not worth meeting someone interesting . . . so work on it by declaring every day, many times a day, that you are capable, that you are a wonderful person, that you speak with confidence, etc.

About the Author

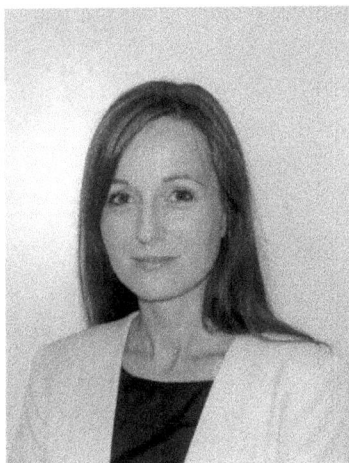

Justine Lamboley is a recognised integrative medicine and energy healing practitioner, a self-empowerment leader, and a positive communication advisor. She is a committed catalyst of change who supports others to achieve optimum health and enjoy happiness in their life.

A former journalist with CNN, BBC, and France 24, Justine was educated at the leading French university, Sciences-Po Paris. She has combined the most powerful secret tools used by successful leaders, healers, and millionaires along with the latest scientific findings in the field of health and well-being to provide a unique expertise in the field of natural health. Justine is dedicated to share these techniques and help people put them into action to live a prosperous and self-fulfilling daily life.

Justine is also a gifted multilingual (French, English, and Arabic) author and speaker who gives conferences about nutrition, health, and well-being. She shares her time between the French Riviera (Nice) and the Middle East (Oman).

Contact

Stay in touch with me to get the latest articles about health and well-being, ask health-related questions, give your feedback, comments, and suggestions.

E-mail: justine.lamboley@haim.academy

Twitter: @justinelamboley

Facebook: I am still resisting re-opening a Facebook account so far...it might change in the future. Meanwhile you can connect to my author page www.facebook.com/JustineLamboley

Website: www.haim.academy

Register with H'AIM (Health And Integrative Medicine), my publishing house, to receive exclusive articles and information about health and happiness. You will also be able to see up-coming workshops and events.

www.haim.academy

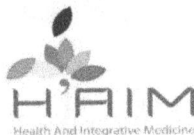

H'AIM
Health And Integrative Medicine

Thank You!

I hope you enjoyed reading this book and are filled with positive energy to see your life change now. I would be very grateful if you take a minute to review Practise Happiness, The Energy of Life.

If you liked the book, I would be very grateful to have your feedback and comments on Amazon or on my website. If you have anything you think I should improve or you did not like about the book, please do send me a personal e-mail and let me know what you think, I make sure I read all e-mails I receive and I am committed to give the best experience to readers, so your comments are valuable to me.

Also if you liked the book, share it with your friends and help spread positive energy! Let them know about how to achieve vibrant health, get good food for the body, mind and spirit, free of negativity, and a life filled with success and happiness!

www.ingramcontent.com/pod-product-compliance
Lightning Source LLC
Chambersburg PA
CBHW070756290326
41931CB00011BA/2039